# FOREWORD

I have gone through the book written by Shri Devendra Vora on Acupressure Therapy (Reflexology), making available simple directions for using the acupressure therapy to preserve one's health and to cure illness if it overtakes one.

The human body is a perfect machine which can regulate itself, provided the natural rules of food, work and rest are observed. When we transgress natural rules, we create toxins in the body, which the body attempts to get rid of. This attempt is considered as disease and is given different names according to different symptoms. If the transgression of rules is set right by natural methods available to every human being, complete cure is possible without any other aid. This is Nature Cure Treatment which includes the following methods :

( 1 ) Fasting as long as necessary and then dieting properly, using enema, mud packs, steam and friction baths.

( 2 ) Using wheat sprouts and their juice along with a raw diet.

( 3 ) Living only on fresh and raw vegetables, to be taken regularly in a proper manner.

( 4 ) Using magnets to cure illness as prescribed in Magneto Therapy.

( 5 ) Adopting Acupressure Therapy which is described in this book in simple language with clear instructions.

( 6 ) Adopting Urine (Auto) Therapy which can cure all illnesses and maintain both mental and physical health.

Every person can use any one or more of these methods according to his conviction and convenience. What is required is faith in the treatment adopted.

I am glad Shri Vora is publishing this important and useful manual on Acupressure Therapy, so that any person who is interested in Natural Treatment can be his own Doctor of Health. I hope this book will be translated into all Indian languages.

Mumbai, Date : 26.4.1982      **–Morarji Desai**

# PREFACE

Though I am at present engaged in international business as per my desire, my second choice was to go in for the medical line. I had an abiding interest in Health Science since my childhood and I used to learn as much as I could about Health Science. My curiosity was amply rewarded in 1977 when I got an opportunity to study Health Science during my tour of the U.S.A. I came to know that Acupressure Therapy was put to test in the U.S.A. and found very useful. I went deep into it and found its roots in India as remote as 5000 years ago. The chart of the soles given in this book is based on the writings of "Sushrut". Acupressure is only an offspring of Nature's own science installed in our body and given as a great boon to mankind. Acupressure therapy was being followed in different forms in different countries and even the Red Indians in the 16th century cured diseases by pressing different points on the patient's soles. Dr. William Fritzgerald and others of the U.S.A. have carried out research on the same and have brought this science to light in the 20th century.

This therapy is capable of solving the present-world health problems and bestowing good health on all in just 10 years.

**From the view point of health the world could be divided into :**

( 1 ) (About 60 %) – those people (including those to be born) who are healthy but liable to catch diseases). With the regular Acupressure treatment, their illness can be prevented.

( 2 ) (About 25 %) – those people who are suffering at present but can be cured without cost with the help of this science and prevented from falling ill again.

( 3 ) (About 15 %) – who require medical help, medicine and/or surgery. There are enough practitioners and hospitals in the world that can take care of these people. Afterwards, they can also be prevented from falling ill, with the use of Acupressure Therapy.

Thus, with proper propagation and teaching of this science, most of the health problems of the world can be solved. This can be done easily as mentioned below :

( 1 ) This therapy should be learnt by the teachers of high schools and professors at the college level and taught as a voluntary subject. These students, in turn, will propagate this therapy not only in their homes but also in the community around during their vacations.

4

( 2 ) Retired teachers, professors, government servants and other educated people can learn it and conduct classes to teach it to others.

( 3 ) The press can greatly assist by regularly publishing articles on various aspects of this therapy and the experiences of their readers.

( 4 ) It can also be propagated through the media like Radio, TV and Cinema.

( 5 ) Philanthropists and charitable organisations, religious-minded people and religious institutions can adopt this as a God-given therapy and work for its propagation.

The huge amount which is being spent on health problems can better be diverted towards better hygiene, better and cheaper supply of nutritious food to the people and thus create a goodwill cycle to bring health and happiness to all.

The World Health Organisation is now giving attention to this therapy. The West has accepted acupuncture. Very soon the world will accept this Health Science which is the mother of Acupuncture, Siatsu or Pointed Pressure Therapy.

Nature's gifts like sunshine, air and water are free and so is this science. Even a child can easily understand and practise it. Any one can practise it himself for his health. Cheap home devices can be used if so desired.

We shall always be grateful to those unknown Rishis or Sages who discovered the points installed in our palms and soles to be pressed for treatment under this therapy and made us aware of these points. We are also grateful to all those who have preserved this science through the centuries and to those who have helped to encourage this science.

These *Rishis* have taught that the body consists of five elements, namely : Earth *(Prithvi)*, Water *(Jal)*, Fire *(Agni)*, Air *(Vayu)*, and Space *(Akash)* and all these are governed by Bio-Electricity or Life Battery. In order to maintain proper balance of these in our body we should take food and drink according to the season. Some foods which are useful in one season can be harmful in another season, e.g. buttermilk and curd are useful in summer but are not advisable in monsoon. Or fresh vegetables which are useful in summer and winter can be a cause of disease in the

5

monsoon, because of excess of water substance and the possibility of the water being polluted in the monsoon. Similarly, the excess of any one of these substances leads to a national health problem e.g., in Japan, cold is very common. It is due to (i) dampness of air (ii) and more water substance contained in their staple food of rice and fish. Incidence of common cold means that Nature wants to throw out excess of water from the body and any attempt to retain it would lead to more diseases. The best cure for the people of Japan is to take food like wheat regularly, have sunbath, drink boiled and lukewarm water, practise more Sun Pranayam and avail themselves of this science. In Afghanistan, there is more fire element in the human body. Dry air, dry fruits and the blazing sun lead to the excess of heat which causes bleeding through the nose. This can be treated by taking more green watery fruits like watermelon, honeydew, etc., and also by avoiding the use of dry fruits in summer and using buttermilk and curd and practising Moon Pranayam.

In this book, on page 120 of fig. 68 I have shown an easy way to find out which eatables/drinks will suit our body. If it is practised regularly, our diet will become most balanced and as such we shall be able to control and cure most of the diseases.

I have only to urge all those who love health to follow Nature and carry out research and accept whatever is found beneficial.

Louis Pasteur's research about germs is a boon to mankind. But in his enthusiasm, he has overlooked the fact that man – human body – is very much superior and is capable of fighting all the germs and throwing them out of the body by creating antibodies. Diseases caused by these germs enter the body through eatables kept in the open and through overripe fruits as well as through drinking polluted water. We can avoid these things. Therefore, the best cure for health is to empower the Human battery – to recharge the organs and endocrine glands through this therapy and maintain proper hygiene. If these instructions of Nature are followed properly, good health can be enjoyed. However, for those already suffering from incurable diseases, drugs or surgery may be used.

I am most grateful to Shri Morarjibhai Desai, the former Prime Minister of India, for taking great interest in this science and encouraging me to write this book and also for blessing me with his 'FOREWORD'.

I am also grateful to all those who have taken great interest in this Health Science and spread it among a large number of people.

Dr. Jullian N. Kenyon, M.D. of U.K. mentions in his book "21 st Century Medicine" that all the therapies based on bio-electricity will prevail in the world. Among all such therapies, Acupressure is the easiest, simplest and the BEST "Do-it-Yourself" therapy. Only this therapy gives prevention, proper diagnosis and cure for A to Z diseases. Till mankind survives, this therapy will be the Therapy of the world".

Dr Andrew Weil, M.D. of U.S.A. in his book "Spontaneous Healing" maintains that our body has a great capacity to heal itself.

We all stand on the shoulders of our predecessors. We are grateful to all of them. This book is a humble effort to explain Nature's science and its technology in a simple way, from a layman's angle in the hope that it will benefit the people at large.

As laymen, we are interested in quick recovery and would not mind using harmless, complementary medicines. As such, the use of such medicines and of some hints of the Pointed Pressure Therapy Siatsu are included in this book. Acupressure therapy has been tried by more than 5 million people in the past five years and in 85 % cases it has succeeded. Nobody has reported any side effects. Several instances can be given here. But the following report of Dr Rahmaney, M.B.B.S. and Homoeopath of Malegaon is very inspiring :

"Women working on hand spinning wheels suffered from cuts in fingertips near the nails made by the thread of the yarn. Infection and then whitlow put them in a very painful condition. Moreover, throbbing pain at night caused sleeplessness and rendered them unable to work during the day to earn their daily bread. And this caused loss of labour for a week or two. Further, the opening of the abscess required dressing for weeks together. Acu- pressure treatment was given to hundreds of such patients and they were taught to do the same at home. Pressure was given on the nearest point or on exactly the same point on the opposite hand. By this treatment patients got relief from pain, had good sleep at night, and within 3 to 5 days it was found that the pus and inflammation had gone and the dead skin got peeled off. Now these women press their tired fingers after every $1\frac{1}{2}$ hour or so. There are no more cuts, there is no more pain. They bless me and I thank Acupressure Therapy".

Similarly, I have cured many patients of Mastitis i.e., pain in breasts after delivery, Appendicitis, stomach pain, B. P., etc. by this Acupressure Therapy.

I request all health-loving people, benevolent institutions and the Government to give a trial to this therapy and propagate it if found useful. The suggestions given in this book for the treatment of various diseases have been found useful and so are given out for the benefit of all the people without any legal liability to myself.

Let us not forget the kind mother Nature in our pursuit of science. In the end I pray that :

**"Welfare be to all the world;**

**May all be interested in helping others;**

**Diseases and misery may perish;**

**And may all the people be Healthy and Happy."**

Now, the revised edition of this book is published. I have added chapters about our body, its working and also Nature's other therapies of Nature Cure, Chromotherapy, Urine Therapy and Biochemic therapy; and many new hypothecations based on my personal examination of over 1,25,000 people. I am grateful to all my readers and the publishers.

**23 – 12 – 1989**                                                    **– Devendra Vora**

Based on my experience, this book is revised again to make it more useful to people.

**30 – 12 – 97**

From the experience of practice for twenty years and personal examination of over 2,00,000 patients, I am revising this book to make it more useful and reliable.

# GALA PUBLISHERS OFFER
## Very useful, low priced health books

1. Health in Your Hands : Volume 1
2. Health in Your Hands : Volume 2
3. Be Your Own Doctor with Acupressure
4. Be Your Own Doctor with Foot Reflexology
5. Be Your Own Doctor with Magnet Therapy
6. Nature Cure for Common Diseases
7. Juice-Diet for Perfect Health
8. Efficacy of Fasting
9. Prevent Heart Disease and Prolong Life
10. From Fat to Fit
11. Backache : Prevention and Cure
12. Diabetes, High Blood Pressure, Without Any Fear
13. Panacea on the Earth : Wheat Grass Juice
14. Vision Training Programme
15. Care of the Eyes
16. Incurable Disease ? Don't Despair
17. Auto-Urine Therapy
18. Be Your Own Doctor Using REIKI
19. Yoga : Yogasanas and Pranayama for Health
20. Holy Basil Tulsi
21. The Pregnancy and Baby-Care Book
22. Homoeopathy for Common Diseases
23. Acupressure Chart
24. Shivambu Geeta
25. Defeat Depression
26. A Unique Remedy for A Hundread Ailments : Fasting
27. Health Aerobic and Beauty
28. Arthritis ? Try Yogasanas
29. Health at Your Fingertips
30. Our Valued Treasure – Our Children

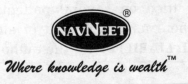

# CONTENTS

After giving treatment on other points, treatment must be given on point No. 26 (kidney).

For children, treatment must also be given on point 38.

(**Note :** Treatment suggested in this book is successfully tried on several patients and so is mentioned here for the benefit of all **WITHOUT ANY LEGAL LIABILITY** for the author.)

# CHAPTER 1

# OUR BODY

Of all kinds of happiness, the best happiness is good health i.e. freedom from any worries about one's body or diseases. That is why we should know more about our body and how to look after it.

According to science the human body appeared on Earth more than 5 million years ago. It is the greatest wonder. It is intriguing to find out which machine of the present machine-age is not placed in our body by the Creator. All these delicate but strong machines can work non-stop even for 100 years and work in unbelievable harmony. **Moreover, this human body is capable of curing any disease.** Acupressure helps the body in this process of CURE and also to maintain all organs and endocrine glands in a proper working order – so that we get PERFECT HEALTH and the possibility of any disease is greatly reduced.

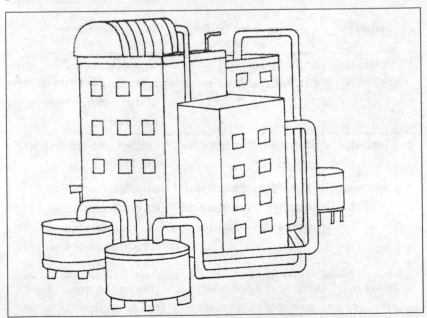

Fig. 1 : Human body is like a modern factory

We can compare our body with the most modern, mobile, airconditioned factory. Its building has a cement concrete structure and is built on pillars – the legs which give it movement also. Its first floor, which is up to diaphragm, accommodates the nutrition producing plant, filteration plant and even sewage plant to throw out wastage – urine and stools. Surprisingly, it has a unique reproduction plant. On the second floor of this human building there is a non-stop pump (Heart) and also air controllers (Lungs). The upper/top floor is dome-shaped and it accommodates the atomic reactor, super-computer and telephone exchange (Brain) which has miles-long, a fastest communication system. And surprisingly, all the different plants work AUTOMATICALLY and in co-ordination. This human factory has the following inbuilt systems in it :

## THE ORGAN SYSTEMS OF THE BODY

| System | Major Organs, Component Tissues, or Cells | Functions |
|---|---|---|
| 1. Skeletal | body bones and cartilage joints. | support, protection, give form and shape to the body; act as levers for movement |
| 2. Muscular | body muscles attached to skeleton. | skilled and gross body movement. |
| 3. Nervous | brain, spinal cord, all peripheral nerves and organs of sensation. | appreciation of environment, co-ordination and direction of activities of body organs |
| 4. Integu- mentary | skin and appendages (hair, nails, glands) | protection against invasion from outside, dehydration, injury and temperature regulation |

| 5. Digestive | mouth, mouth cavity, pharynx, oesophagus, stomach, intestines, anus, liver, pancreas and salivary glands | ingestion, digestion absorption of nutrients and ejection of residues |
|---|---|---|
| 6. Respiratory | nose, nasal cavities, larynx, trachea, lungs, (bronchi and bronchioles), lungs | take in oxygen; expel carbon dioxide; acid-base regulation |
| 7. Circulatory | heart, artery, veins, capillary, blood and blood vessels | transport of nurtients, cell products to and wastes from all parts of the body |
| 8. Immune | white blood cells, certain cells of bone marrow, lymph nodes, spleen, etc. | defence against foreign cells, micro-organisms, parasites and viruses |
| 9. Urinary (excretory) | kidneys, ureters, urinary bladder and urethra | regulation of blood composition; formation and elimination of urine |
| 10. Reproductive | **Female :** ovaries, fallopian tubes, uterus, vagina, external genitalia, mammary glands **Male :** testes, vas deferens, seminal vesicles, prostate and external genitalia | production of sex cells (ova, sperm); hormone production |
| 11. Lymphatic (lymph vascular) | Lymph nodes, nodules, vessels, thymus and spleen | return of fluid to circulation; clearing of dead cells from body, part of immune system |

**Skeleton :** The frame of a fully developed body looks like the skeleton shown in the picture here. It is composed of 206 bones, which are of different types. The skull bones are devised to give maximum protection to the brain–the atomic reactor, super-computer and telephone exchange of our body, vertebrae spine bones give protection to the sciatic nerves–the main cable, cage of ribs give protection to the vital lungs and heart, and bones of hands and legs give movement. This frame of bones looking like a cement-concrete structure of a building is made mainly of calcium and phosphorous and small amounts of a few mineral compounds.

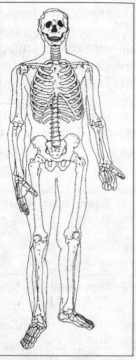

Fig. 2 : Skeleton – cement concrete structure

Many of these bones are hollow inside where the most vital new red cells are generated. So when blood passes through these bones, red cells get mixed into it. That is why when a patient suffers from blood cancer, the bone marrow is also damaged. This in turn leads to less production of red blood cells and this vicious cycle leads to fatal consequences.

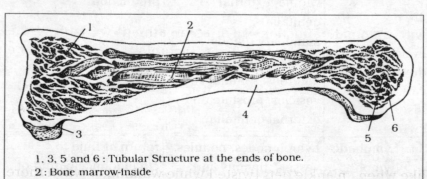

1, 3, 5 and 6 : Tubular Structure at the ends of bone.
2 : Bone marrow-inside
4 : Hollow-inside

Fig. 3 : Structure of a bone

These bones contain inorganic chemicals like calcium, phosphorous, iron, etc. which make these bones hard; and also organic chemicals which produce red blood cells. These bones complete their growth before 20 to 23 years and so after this age height does not increase.

**Muscles :** (They are like the brick work with plaster inside.) The bones and their joints are covered with muscles. There is a network of muscles in the body and it weighs more than 50 % of the body's weight. Muscles are fibrous tissues that produce movement in the body. They are secured to the bones by cords called the tendons. You can easily see the tendons at work by moving your hand and noticing where these cords move underneath the skin. The bones of moving joints are secured together by fibres called ligaments and soft pads of cartilage. They act as cushions where the bones move over each other. Muscles work in groups, so in order to move a limb certain muscles contract and pull on the tendons, thus moving the bone, while compensating muscles stretch to keep the movement steady. Muscles are mainly of two types : voluntary and involuntary. The voluntary muscles work as per our will and are mainly concerned with movements of limbs. Involuntary muscles are found in the blood vessels, in the iris of the eye, trachea, food pipe, heart, diaphragm, etc. in the body. In short, the voluntary muscles carry out controlled movements, while the involuntary muscles with their slow rhythmic movements are concerned with automatic functions such as breathing, working of the heart, food digestion, etc. These voluntary muscles can be developed and made strong by exercises. Heavy exercises can build up these muscles, but in that case, these muscles lose their suppleness. But yogic exercises, walking, swimming, etc. give suppleness and tone to these muscles.

If there is undue pressure on these joints and ligaments, like when an ankle gets twisted while walking or when there is a fall, there is a sprain in these joints and ligaments. In such cases, the pain subsides with rest, and with the application of hot/cold packs. The affected part should be covered with elastic bands.

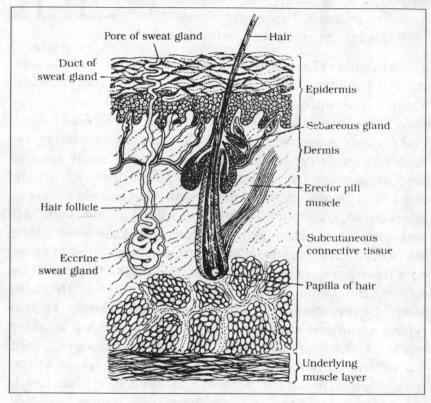

**Fig. 4 : Seven layers of skin**

**Skin :** It is like an outside plaster of a building. The framework of bones, skeleton, muscles and fats, are covered with skin which has seven layers, but only 1.5 millimeter thick and it is porous. It has its outer layer with sensory glands which impart to us its sense of touch; the real skin and respiration glands. They are connected by both types of afferent and efferent nerves which take sensations of coldness, heat, softness, hardness, pressure, etc. to the brain and bring back the orders from the brain. The skin protects the muscles and fats of the body. It also prevents bacteria from entering the body. Moreover, many toxins are thrown out of the body through the skin, thus serving as a blood purifier. It helps the removal of certain salts of the body through perspiration. It controls the temperature of the body and prevents cold from entering the body in cold season and throws out heat in the hot season through perspiration. The hair on the skin also assist in controlling the temperature of the body.

Surprisingly, even though the skin is thin and delicate, it is very strong and elastic.

**Digestive System :** (Nutritive material manufacturing wonderful chemical plant of the body.)

For the working of the body and nutrition, the organs, muscles and other tissues require blood. Pure blood is formed from the food and drink we take and digest. Our digestive system consists of mouth, buccal cavity, oesophagus, stomach, intestines (small and big), ileocaecal valve, pancreas, liver, etc.

**Mouth :** This is the opening of the system through which food and drink enter the system.

**Buccal Cavity :** This is the hollow space behind the teeth where the food is chewed with the help of teeth. Saliva is secreted from the salivary glands. This mixes with the food and helps in the digestion of sugars. Proper chewing of food at least 12-15 times is most necessary. Talks should be avoided while eating – instead, light music could be played.

**Oesophagus (Gullet) :** Normally this remains closed, but when food is forced into it, it directs the food downwards automatically with special movement called peristalsis. This food is pushed into the stomach.

**Stomach (Mixer) (Point No. 27) :** When the food enters the stomach, it secretes digestive juices like pepsin and renin which help in the digestion of proteins. The churning of the food and mixing of the digestive juices goes on for about 4 hours. Then the semidigested and liquified food finds its way into the duodenum through the pyloric valve.

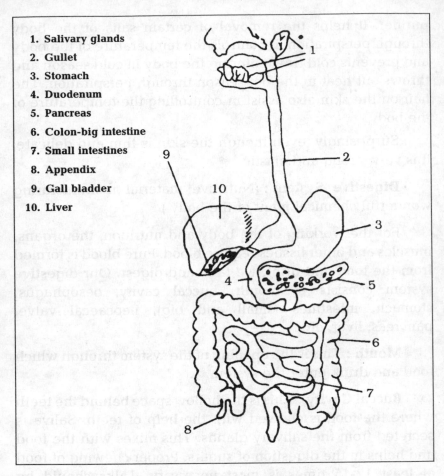

1. Salivary glands
2. Gullet
3. Stomach
4. Duodenum
5. Pancreas
6. Colon-big intestine
7. Small intestines
8. Appendix
9. Gall bladder
10. Liver

**Fig. 5 : Digestive organs**

In order to enable the stomach to function efficiently, one should not overload it with food more than necessary, so that it can expand and contract properly. Moreover, one should make a habit of not eating between two meals and to give 9 to 10 hours of rest to the stomach at night. "To live long and healthy eat only when you are very hungry." said Sir M. Visvesvarayya, eminent engineer, educationist and Bharat Ratna award winner, who lived for 101 years.

**Small Intestine (Point No. 19) :** It is about twenty-three feet i.e. seven metres long tube. The anterior (about nine inch) part is called duodenum. The bile juice created by the liver (Point No. 23) and stored in the gall bladder (Point No. 22) and pancreatic juice are poured into the duodenum where it mixes with the food. Jejunum, the middle part of the small intestine is about seven to eight feet long. The last part is called Ilium and is about fifteen to sixteen feet long. Digestive juices secreted here get mixed with the food and help in the digestion. The bile is alkaline in nature. It neutralizes and renders the semi-digested acidic food coming from the stomach, alkaline; so as to allow the pancreatic enzymes to act. Bile juice also helps the fat to be emulified and made soluble for easy digestion. Most of the food is digested in the small intestine and broken down into simpler products like amino acids, monosaccharides like glucose, monoglycerides and free fatty acids which are absorbed in the small intestine. These absorbed juices are turned into blood by spleen. The unabsorbed residue goes into the large intestines through ileocaecal valve (Point No. 21). It is the world's best sewage system. The necessary amount of water and certain salts are absorbed here. This large intestine consists of the caecum (with the appendix) and the colon which ends into rectum. Depending on their position, parts of the colon are named as ascending colon, traverse colon, descending colon and the sigmoid colon. Inflammation of the colon is known as Colitis. It may be noted that if the food is properly digested and liquid intake is sufficient, the stool is properly formed-soft and nearly odourless.

**Appendix (Point No. 21) :** It is a worm shaped tube arising from the caecum. It is about four inches long and has no special function, but it often gets inflamed due to accumulation of decaying faecal matter or worms lodged inside it. It causes severe pain and vomitting. This can be corrected with Acupressure treatment [(Change in diet-(say green juices and fruit juices), and surgery can be avoided.)]

**Pancreas (Point No. 25) :** It is a digestive – an exocrine gland; however as it produces insulin, it is also called an endocrine gland. Its digestive juices help in digestion of carbohydrates, proteins and fats. It creates insulin which assists the body in maintaining of sugar level of blood. It is likely that whenever energy is required by the body as demanded by adrenal gland to do some action quickly; the insulin producing parts of pancreas slows down its process and allows more sugar/glucose = energy to go to the necessary parts of the body. Now if this process is repeatedly continued due to excitement over functioning of adrenal gland the pancreas slows down its process of creating enough insulin and over a period of few years becomes sluggish; so the control of sugar/glucose level in the body slows down and a stage is reached where diabetes sets in. Therefore, for those people who are not overweight but have diabetes, should control adrenal and cure excess excitedness and worries and activate the pancreas to cure the diabetes. Thus, if adequate insulin is not produced by the pancreas, the result is diabetes. However, its overworking leads to more consumption of sugar/glucose and leads to low B.P., migraine, headache, etc.

**Liver (Point No. 23) :** Our body has a reactor-producing energy and heat. Our body requires a cooling system to control this heat. This is Liver. Its working can be compared with the working of the radiator of a car. It produces bile juice which is stored in gall bladder (Point No. 22) and from there, whenever necessary, it is poured into the duodenum-part of small intestine and turns the acidic semi-liquid food into alkaline. **Now, if the liver does not function properly and produce sufficient bile and if there is no free flow of this stored bile from gall bladder into the small intestine, acidity in the digestive system increases. This in turn leads to excess heat in the body.** On the one hand more acidity in the digestive system leads to gases, burning sensation in the stomach and in gullet, weakening the gums and the teeth, and later on leading to ulcer in the intestines and the mouth. On the other hand, **production of excess heat in the body becomes the root cause of cold due to heat; disturbs the functioning of the eyes, one of the root causes and it is also that necessitates the use of spectacles,** also it makes the semen, ova thinner – leading to early ejaculation and discharge in sleep for men and also to Leukorrhea in women; it also leads to problems of skin, falling of hair and is one of the main causes of Jaundice. Such a vicious cycle also leads to short-temperedness.

The proper functioning of liver is most vital and hence it is the biggest gland in the body. Moreover, it stores fats, minerals and vitamins. It converts sugar into Glycogen and vice-versa and stores it. Moreover, liver removes toxins and destroys unwanted by-products. Further, it converts cholesterol into bile.

Thus, it will be observed that as proper functioning of many organs of the body depends upon proper functioning of the liver. The quality of life is rightly said to depend upon the liver. However, its functioning is disturbed by excess heat inside the body. Such an excess heat in the body is created by less functioning of liver and also due to cobalt and Infra-Red rays, heat producing anti-biotic drugs, drugs which disturb the proper functioning of liver and also due to the exposure to outside heat. In all these cases, it is utmost necessary to take treatment (shown later on in this book) to reduce excess heat in the body.

Working of liver is controlled by adrenal gland (Point No. 28).

**Respiratory System :** As the body requires food for nutrition, it requires oxygen for energy. For any type of work to be done, the body requires oxygen which helps in producing energy from the stored food materials. Th **oxygen is of prime importance, because if it is not sup**

**to the brain for more than three minutes, the brain stops functioning.**

When the air enters the nose, it is filtered and moistened before it enters the lungs (Point No. 30). Here the impure blood is sent by the heart. The blood in the capillaries of the lungs absorbs oxygen from the inhaled air and release impurities like carbondioxide, hydrogen etc. which are exhaled out. The purified blood is sent back to the heart from where it is pumped into the body and thus oxygen is supplied to all the organs *(see figs. 6 & 7).*

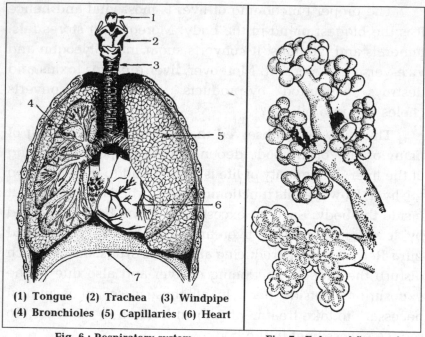

(1) Tongue    (2) Trachea    (3) Windpipe
(4) Bronchioles (5) Capillaries (6) Heart

Fig. 6 : Respiratory system                Fig. 7 : Enlarged figure of
                                            bronchioles/capillaries

For the efficient working of the lungs, the passage has to be clear and big enough to allow a two-way traffic for the fresh air to come into the lungs and carbon dioxide to go out. If these walls get covered with cold-phlegm, this free flow of ingoing and outgoing air becomes difficult and causes breathlessness.

The capacity of the lungs should be fully developed so that it can purify the blood and free it from all toxins. This can be done with breathing exercises, pranayam, swimming and running. Easy methods of pranayam are shown in chapter 5 of this book.

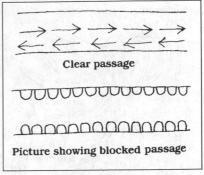

Fig. 8

The air to be breathed in, must be as pure as far as possible. People working in congested cities, workshops, chemical, rubber, tobacco factories where the air is polluted must make it a practice to go out from time to time in the open and do pranayam and revitalise this important respiratory system which occupies the maximum space in our body. The lungs are a very vital organ supplying oxygen to all the parts of our body and the brain. If this oxygen supply is not maintained for more than three minutes, the brain stops functioning. **The more the air we breathe in and retain, the better it is for our vitality.**

**Circulatory Systems – Heart :** Point No. 36 (a non-stop pump). It is a hollow muscle and because of rhythmic contraction (systole) and expansion (diastole) the blood is collected and pumped to the whole body. It has four compartments; when the heart expands, impure blood comes into upper right compartment known as the right auricle. At that time, the purified blood also comes into 2nd upper left compartment known as the left auricle. From there, the impure blood passes through the valve into the right ventricle – the lower right compartment and the purified blood passes through the valve into the lower left compartment known as left ventricle. Now, when the heart contracts the impure blood is pumped into lungs and the purified blood is sent to the whole body *(See fig. 10)*.

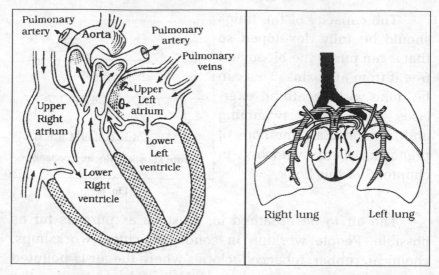

Fig. 9 : Heart with four          Fig. 10 : Purification of
compartments                      blood in lungs

For a sedentary adult person, the heart throbs about 72 times in a minute while for persons doing manual work exercise, it throbs for about 50 to 60 times – thus less work for the heart and so less danger of heart attack. This is the main reason why running, swimming, exercises, yoga, etc. are advised. Moreover, in a minute about five litres of blood flows from the heart. The heart is like a closed fist and weighs about 250 gms in a female and 300 gms in a male.

In order that the heart can function properly, the outside wall muscles also require oxygen, blood circulation and electricity. It can be revitalised with rest, Acupressure treatment and gold charged water.

**Blood :** Out of the extract sucked from small intestines the liquid juice is turned into blood by the spleen (Point No. 37). It then goes into the heart from where it is pumped into the whole body providing nutrition and oxygen to all its cells. Carbon-toxins are sucked by the blood and brought back to the heart which in turn pumps blood into the lungs for purification before it is pumped again into the body.

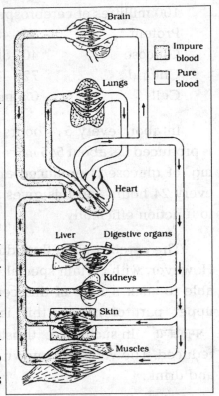

Blood also passes through the kidney (Point No. 26), where it is filtered and the toxins are then passed out by the kidney to the bladder (Point No. 18) and then thrown out of the body. If the lungs do not function properly, it will not be able to suck all the carbon toxins from the blood. This will, thus,

Fig. 11 : Circulation of blood

put an excess burden on the kidney rendering them unfit to filter all the toxins from the blood and then throw them out of our system. The unfiltered toxins are thrown out of the system through the skin and are known as skin problems.

**Cerebrospinal Fluid :** When the blood goes into the head, it passes through 1st and 2nd ventricle, where cerebro-spinal fluid is extracted from the blood. This is a very vital life juice – nectar of life. Yogis call it Nectar (अमृत). This cerebrospinal fluid passes through the brain and goes down in the spinal cord up to prostate gland and keeps the neuron motors working.

100 millitres of cerebrospinal fluid contains :

Protein                15 – 45 mg
Glucose                40 – 50 mg
Chloride               720 – 750 mg
Cells                  0.5 mg + lymphocytes, etc.

In about every 5 1/2 hours 125 ml of cerebrospinal fluid is produced i.e. about 545 ml cerebrospinal fluid and 200 – 250 mg. of glucose is produced and consumed by the body in every 24 hours and this gives vital energy to all the organs to function efficiently.

The cerebrospinal fluid does not get mixed with blood. However, with certain special yogic exercises, the yogis are able to suck a little of this cerebrospinal fluid through the upper part of mouth – this is called – drinking of Nectar "अमृतक्रिया". In such cases, thrist and hunger are considerably reduced. The yogis are known to live on a minimum of food and drink.

**Root cause of High B. P. :** This cerebrospinal fluid enters the 3rd ventricle from the bottom, rises upward and then goes into the central nervous system through a small outlet. Now due to the excess common salt = (Sodium Chloride) in cerebrospinal fluid or may be due to .tension, the tiny hair like cells in the valve of outlet, get stiff and hamper the proper flow of cerebrospinal

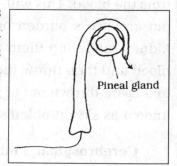

Pineal gland

Fig. 12 : Picture showing 3rd Ventricle and Pineal gland below the small outlet

fluid into the central nervous system. So, the pressure – (force to send the cerebrospinal fluid upward) increases in the 3rd ventricle causing what is known as high blood pressure (High B.P.) The pineal gland situated under the valve gets damaged when B. P. increases and thus its working is impaired. As this gland controls all the other glands, their working is also damaged leading to problems in the body. So, the best way to control high B. P. is (1) to control the Pineal and other endocrine glands through Acupressure as an immediate cure, (2) for long term cure reduce common salt intake in food (one can take rock salt i.e. potassium chloride) and (3) empower the system by drinking two glasses of gold/silver/copper charged water, reduced from four glasses.

**Root cause of Low B. P. :** Low blood pressure is caused by the over functioning of Pancreas which reduces the sugar-glucose level in the blood; in turn the level of glucose content in cerebrospinal fluid is also reduced, thereby the supply of energy to the vital brain and motor neurons is also reduced. Consequently, the body becomes weak. It is, therefore, necessary to give extra glucose to the patient by giving him hot tea/coffee, milk with more sugar as an immediate treatment and control pancreas as a long term cure.

**Excretory (Urinating) System :** Everyday out of 175 litres of blood filtered by kidney, about 1.5 litre of waste is sent to the bladder from where it is periodically thrown out as urine.

**Reproductive System :** This has a great function of reproduction through which human race continues. Suprisingly male and female parts of the human body machine are capable of producing the same type of humans and also giving one of the great joys of life. It is therefore, necessary to take proper care of its organs and keep them hygienically clean and not to waste semen and ova. When puberty is reached around the age of 12 to 14 years in girls, their menstruation cycle starts and 14 to 16 years in boys, when they start growing moustache and beard on the face.

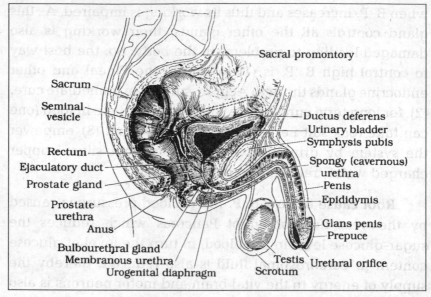

**Fig. 13 : Reproductive organs of a male**

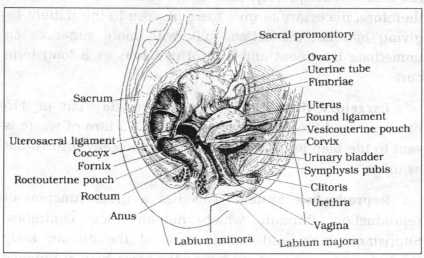

**Fig. 14 : Reproductive organs of a female**

**Immune System :** Our body has an excellent inbuilt protective system which creates antibodies through the creation of white cells and throws out the dead cells through Lymph glands (Point No. 16). This is a unique defence system always active against intrusion by foreign cells, micro-organisms, parasites and viruses.

In our body – a mobile factory – there are several delicate but powerful instruments. These are interrelated through the brain. These organs of five senses of **Touch (Skin); Smell (Nose); Taste (Tongue); Hearing (Ears)** and **Vision (Eyes) enable us to learn and enjoy Life.**

**Touch :** We have seen the working of the skin through which we feel and get to know about things around us.

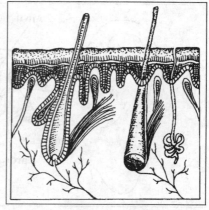

Fig. 15 : Skin

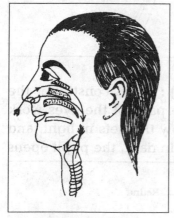

Fig. 16 : Nose

**Nose :** Over and above breathing through the two nostrils and maintaining the equilibrium of heat in the body, the nose enables us to smell.

**Taste :** The tongue enables us to get all types of tastes – one of the best experiences in life. It also controls our speech.

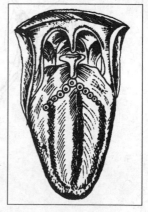

Fig. 17 : Tongue

**Hearing (Ears) (Point No. 31) :** It is a most intricate and profound sound system that enables us to acquire knowledge by hearing. Only when we can hear, can we speak. The combination of hearing and speech is like an accordian (musical instrument) placed in our throat so that one can sing the finest tunes.

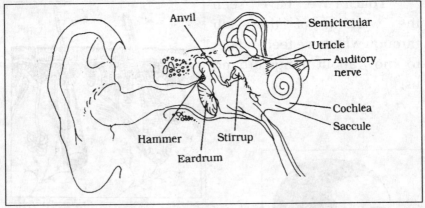

Fig. 18 : Ears

**Vision (Eyes) (Point No. 35) :** They constitute the camera and colour projector. All the parts of the eyes work together. The cornea is like a window that lets in light, and the iris controls the amount of light. In dark, the pupil opens

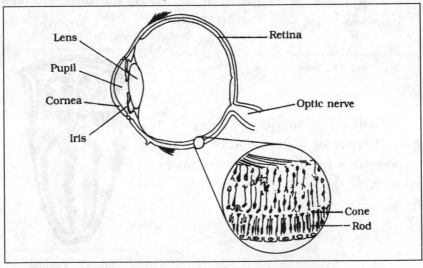

Fig. 19 : Eyes

wide to let the light come in and in bright, it becomes smaller. The lens is a tissue that adjusts like a focus. The retina is the lining of the inside of the eyes which has many nerve endings. They react when light falls on the retina which is filled with small cells called rods and cones. Cones are sensitive to colour. Rods are not sensitive and enable us to see in less light. The optic nerve is the pathway to the brain. It carries signals and nutrition to the eyes. The eyes get the electric current from the brain.

**Central Nervous System (Communication System– Telephone Exchange) :** This consists of the brain, brain stem, sciatic nerve and miles of nerves coming out of this sciatic nerve spreading all over the body.

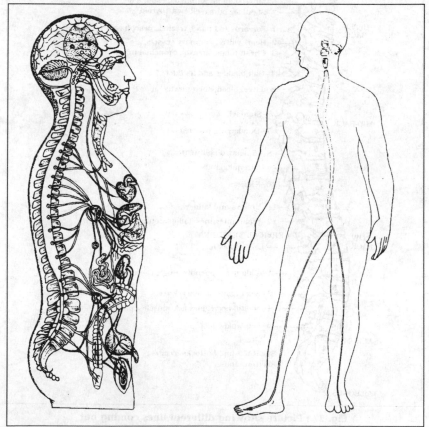

Fig. 20 : Central nervous system          Fig. 21 : Sciatic nerve

It may be noted that below the brain – the telephone exchange – a quarter inch thick sciatic nerve (can be called as the cable cord of telephone system) passes down through the vertebrae of spine going up to the coccyx, gets divided into two and then goes all the way down to both the legs and finally to the toes as shown in fig. 21.

It will be observed that the small nerves coming out of the spinal cord – sciatic nerve – are joined to different organs

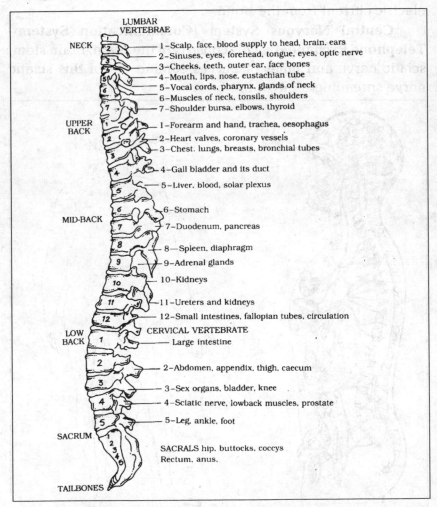

LUMBAR VERTEBRAE

NECK
1 – Scalp, face, blood supply to head, brain, ears
2 – Sinuses, eyes, forehead, tongue, eyes, optic nerve
3 – Cheeks, teeth, outer ear, face bones
4 – Mouth, lips, nose, eustachian tube
5 – Vocal cords, pharynx, glands of neck
6 – Muscles of neck, tonsils, shoulders
7 – Shoulder bursa, elbows, thyroid

UPPER BACK
1 – Forearm and hand, trachea, oesophagus
2 – Heart valves, coronary vessels
3 – Chest, lungs, breasts, bronchial tubes
4 – Gall bladder and its duct
5 – Liver, blood, solar plexus

MID-BACK
6 – Stomach
7 – Duodenum, pancreas
8 – Spleen, diaphragm
9 – Adrenal glands
10 – Kidneys
11 – Ureters and kidneys
12 – Small intestines, fallopian tubes, circulation

LOW BACK
CERVICAL VERTEBRATE
Large intestine
2 – Abdomen, appendix, thigh, caecum
3 – Sex organs, bladder, knee
4 – Sciatic nerve, lowback muscles, prostate
5 – Leg, ankle, foot

SACRUM
SACRALS hip, buttocks, coccys
Rectum, anus.

TAILBONES

**Fig. 22 : Picture showing different lines coming out of vertebrae connected with different organs**

in the middle and front part of the body as shown in fig. 20 & 22. If there is any disturbance in or damage to the spinal cord, the flow of electricity to the connecting organs is hindered. If, for example, vertebra no. 4 is subdued, it impairs speech and causes stammering. When treatment is given on this point of vertebra no. 4, the problem of stammering is cured.

Similarly, if due to cold, the point on the sciatic nerve between vertebra no. 6 and 8 is damaged, it transmits pain to the muscles around the heart and this indication is mistaken as a heart problem.

Thus, it is very vital that the sciatic nerve works properly. For this reason sitting erect is necessary and the following daily exercise will be found very useful.

In the morning stand erect keeping the legs 12/15 inches apart. Raise the hands and try to go backward from the waist as much as possible inhaling at the same time. Then come forward and bend from the waist with extended hands while exhaling at the same time. It will be observed that due to improper sitting and sleeping practice, the sciatic nerve is contracted and it may not be possible to touch the ground.

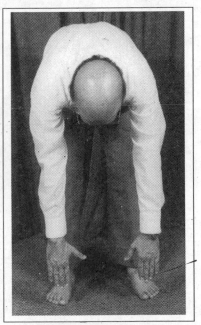

Fig. 23 : How to strech spinal cord

However, when this exercise is repeated, you will be surprised to observe that not only are you able to touch the ground but even go further touching behind the legs. Thus, the spinal cord gets fully stretched and flow of energy is ensured all over the organs.

It is observed that due to the unexpected jerks and lifting of heavy things, cold, wearing of high heeled shoes, etc. the sciatic nerve gets damaged, causing pain in the legs from waist to toes, knees, etc. There is no damage to vertebrae and so the root cause is not detected even in X-rays. However, when pressed on the points of sciatic nerve; as shown in fig. 42 (a) & (b); pain will be felt. After the treatment on the points of sciatic nerve in both the legs, all pain in the legs including knee pain will subside.

———

# CHAPTER 2

# BRAIN : THE ATOMIC REACTOR– BIO-ELECTRICITY

**Brain :** It is the atomic reactor; supercomputer and also telephone exchange of our body. It is the most important part of our central nervous system. Being of great importance, it is protected by the skull and also kept floating in the cerebrospinal fluid. It consists of :

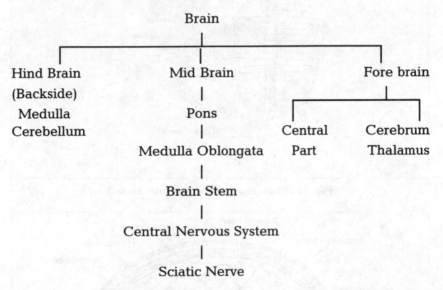

(Popularly known as the Spinal Cord up to lower lumbar & as the Sciatic Nerve from Coccyx up to toes)

**The Cerebellum (Small Brain) :** It is a bundle of nerves like an armature dynamo in a car. When blood passes through it, electricity is produced. The positive current is sent to the brain through the first ventricle and the negative current through the second ventricle. These positive and negative currents recharge the brain cells–the battery of the body and thus keep the motor neurons working. It controls and regulates the unconscious internal activities of the body.

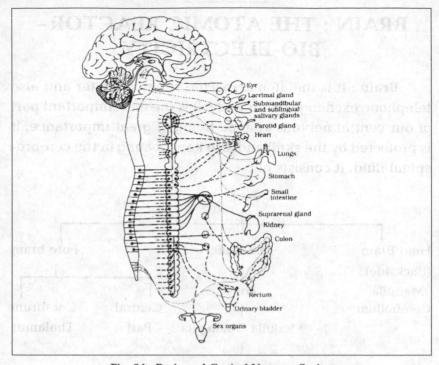

**Fig. 24 : Brain and Central Nervous System**

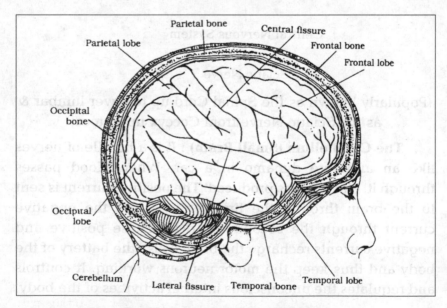

**Fig. 25 : Inside of Cerebrum (big brain)**

Moreover, it coordinates the muscular movements while walking and running and maintains posture and equilibrium of the body. Till birth, all the activities are controlled by the small brain. After birth, its control is taken over by the big brain – the cerebrum.

**The Cerebrum (Big Brain) :** It is the supercomputer. All the knowledge gathered through the five senses, is passed on to the big brain through afferent nerves and this information is analysed on the basis of past knowledge and experience and necessary orders are prepared and passed on to the required organs through efferent nerves. This Cerebrum is made of two large hemispheres each containing different sets of nerves centres. The right side of the brain controls the left side of the body while the left side of the brain controls the right side of the body. There are about 20,000 chips in this supercomputer but we hardly use 10 % of the same. It is said that even for a great scientist like Albert Einstein, only 15 % of his brain was functioning.

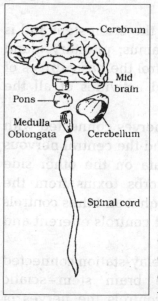

Fig. 26

| Part of the Central Nervous System | Controlling activities |
|---|---|
| Frontal lobe | Judgement and reason |
| Parietal lobe | Movement and senses |
| Occipital lobe | Vision |
| Cerebellum | Muscle coordination |
| Temporal lobe | Speech and hearing |
| Medulla | Autonomic activities, such as breathing and heartbeat. |
| Pons | PH level and death |

From the thalamus all the senses are controlled, through the cerebral cortex, which consists of millions of grey matter and millions of cells of white matter inside and which in turn carry messages to and fro *(See figure 27)*.

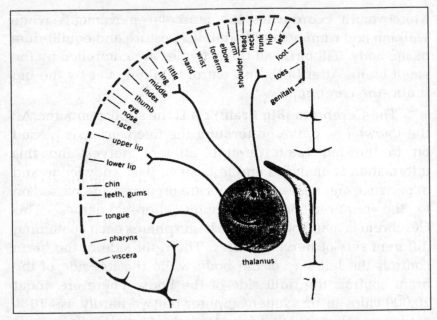

**Fig. 27 : Cortex and its control over various organs of the body**

**Brain stem** consists of midbrain, pons and medula oblongata.

**Midbrain :** It is the upper part of the brain stem and is composed of the hypothalamus, thalamus, pituitary gland and limbic system. Together they control the basic drives of hunger, thirst, body temperature and activities of all the endocrine glands.

**Pons :** It has a set of 12 pairs of nerves connected with the small and big brain on one side and the central nervous system through the medulla oblongata on the other side working like a relay station. It absorbs toxins from the cerebrospinal fluid which passes through it and thus controls the PH level of the body and death. It controls efferent and afferent nerves.

**Medulla Oblongata :** It is also a relay-station connected with pons on one side and the brain stem – sciatic nerve – spinal cord on the other. It controls the nerves of automatic activities such as breathing and heartbeat. And so any damage to it results in immediate death.

**Spinal Cord (Sciatic Nerve) :** As mentioned in chapter 1; It is about 1/4 inch thick cord extending from the brain stem and going down to the coccyx where it gets divided and extends up to the end of the toes. It is also covered with three meninges and also by cerebrospinal fluid. It is made of 31 bundles of nerves which consist the both sensory and motor nerve fibres and carry out impulses to and from the brain. Upper part of the spinal cord is called **Peripheral nervous system** consisting of (1) **somatic system** which controls the skeletal muscles and receives sensory information from the skin, muscles and (2) **automatic system** which controls the involuntary working of the glands, the heart, the blood vessels and linings of stomach and intestines. This automatic nervous system is subdivided into the sympathetic and the parasympathetic which are antagonistic in their action. While the sympathetic nerve system

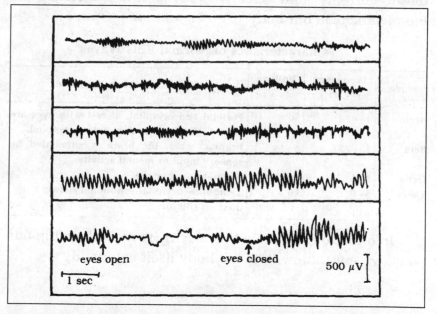

eyes open          eyes closed          500 μV

1 sec

Fig. 28 : Normal EEG patterns from different regions of the cortex. Alpha waves pre-dominate in parietal and occipital areas; beta waves in precentral area. Alpha waves are blocked when eyes are opened.

stimulates the activities of the connecting organs through tissues and gangalia the parasympathetic system brings these organs back to normal.

The body functions automatically as long as the vital organs get nutrition and oxygen through the blood for which the proper functioning of the lungs, heart and digestive system is absolutely necessary. Moreover, the controller of these organs i. e., the brain and central nervous system get nutrition through the cerebrospinal fluid. **However, the whole body becomes listless when there is no supply of power – energy – electricity – pran – chetana life current in it.** Through long and sustained research, it has been found that there are three types of electric currents – Alpha, Beta and Gama (सत्त्व – रजस् – तमस्) which are produced in the brain cells. The picture no. 28 on page 39 shows the EEG patterns of these currents and clearly proves the existence of Bio-electricity in our body.

### Characteristics of Normal EEG Waves

| Wave | Frequency sec (H$_z$) | Voltage (μ V) | Where and When Recorded |
|---|---|---|---|
| Alpha | 10 – 12 | 50 | Parietal and occipital, at rest with eyes are closed. The brain is alert but unoccupied. |
| Beta | 13 – 25 | 5 – 10 | Frontal, when the brain is stimulated by sensory input or mental activity |
| Delta | 1 – 5 | 20 – 200 | Sleep, brain damage |
| Theta | 5 – 8 | 10 | Temporal – occipital, emotional stress; noxious stimuli |

In order to know how this electricity is produced in our body, we must know how the body itself is formed.

**Reproduction System :** When there is a union – intercourse between a male and a female, semen containing about 4 to 5,00,000 spermatozoa is discharged by the male organ into the vagina and only when a sperm is successful in entering the egg of the female, it creates an atomic explosion – the child is conceived.

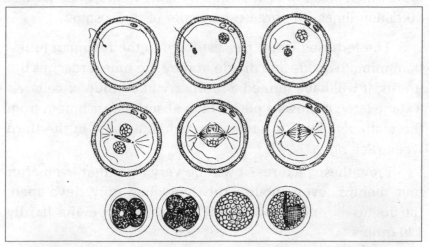

Fig. 29 : Picture showing entering of sperm into egg and multiplication

The ovum of a female is like minus (– – –) electricity and when a spermatozoa which is like (+) positive electricity enters into it, a battery cell is created – produced – as shown below :

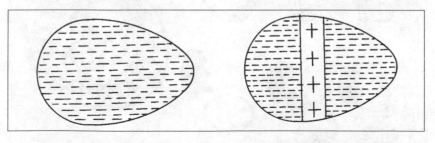

Ovum – Negative electricity          Sperm – Positive electricity

Fig. 30

This fertilised egg then goes on dividing into two and four – thus becomes a quadruplicate and afterwards goes on dividing in quadruplicates only–thus our body has a 4 cylinder electricity producing atomic reactor–battery. The size of this quadruplicate cell is so small that it can be seen with electron microscope but later on it develops into a full sized body of about 60 to 66 inches in height and 60 to 70 kilos which means an expansion by more than 600 crores i. e. 60 billion times–the greatest wonder of the cosmos.

The fertilised ovum passes down to the fallopian tube – beginning to divide and divide and by the time it reaches the uterus, it will have formed a mulberry like group of cells. At a stage later, it grows a placenta to absorb nourishment from the mother's blood. It passes the fish like stage in the third week *(See fig. 31)*.

From these pictures, it will be very clear that even after four months, even though the body has fully developed, the foetus is only about eight inches and weighs hardly 120 grams.

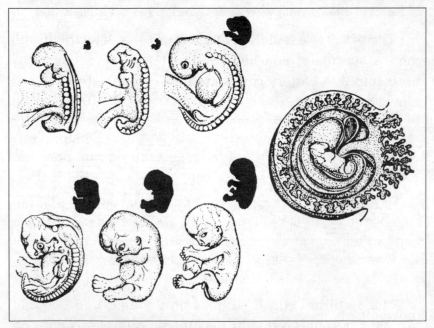

**Fig. 31 : Development of foetus in womb**

It is, therefore, extremely necessary for a pregnant woman to take calcium and other minerals in sufficient quantity for the proper development of the foetus. This calcium is available in milk, banana, green vegetables and fruits. However, this calcium and minerals should be properly digested. Digestion of calcium is controlled by Thyroid/Parathyroid glands and so their proper working

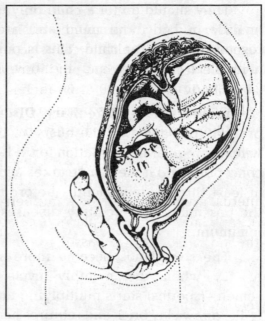

Fig. 32 : Picture of 16 week – foetus fully developed

is utmost necessary during pregnancy; so that the child develops properly and get strong bones. Therefore, the proper functioning of thyroid – parathyroid glands is of prime necessity.

Moreover, the proper development of the foetus in the mother's womb and of the child later on, depends upon the union of the sperm with the egg; so it is of utmost importance that this sperm should be strong and the egg as pure and healthy as possible.

It is really surprising that we take great care in planting a seed – the earth is ploughed – cleared of weeds, stones etc; made softer by watering or by rain and then the best of seed is sown in a proper season. However, while planting a human body, no such care is taken and is just left to an accident. It is the bounden duty of a newly married couple to have full knowledge of the body – the human reproduction system and of the birth of a child besides, of course, child care.

They should go for a child only when both of them are healthy in body and mind and are willing to take the responsibility of the child. This is possible when the girl is more than 18 years and the boy is over 21 – preferably 24 years or more.

**Prevention of Hereditary Diseases :** If the semen is properly preserved by the husband till marriage and if the wife has regular menstruation for at least seven times before conception and if the couple takes acupressure treatment for at least three to four months before the child is conceived, the possibility of hereditary diseases can be reduced to a minimum.

The sex glands become more active around the age of 12, when the monthly cycle starts in girls and semen – (sperms) starts multiplying and maturing in boys. It is like a raw clay brick and requires heat treatment. It is worth noting that semen is not stored anywhere in the body but it becomes syndrome of the body and can be seen as pure white half moons in the nails *(See fig. 33)*.

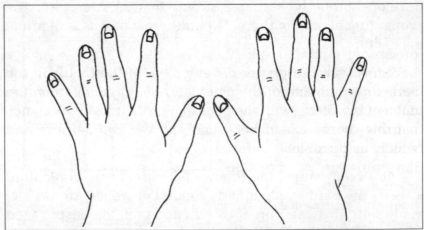

Fig. 33 : Picture showing white half moons in the nails

If precious semen (वीर्य) and (रज) ova are not wasted till the age of 24 in male and 18 in female, this syndrome becomes powerful and strong, so as to protect the body for a lifetime. It may be noted that out of about 40 kilos of food we digest only one litre of blood is formed and out of one litre of blood only a few drops of semen are formed in 49 days in a sequence of seven steps of (1) Liquid (2) Blood (3) Fat (4) Muscles (5) Bones (6) Bone-marrow and (7) Semen.

This clearly shows that if due to any reason this process stops, the body starts putting on more fat. Moreover, blood or semen cannot be produced in a laboratory.

After sperms are created, it takes another 74 days to get them redoubled as shown in the figure 34.

**AIDS :**

Due to excessive abuse of sex, when the level of semen goes down the process of doubling semen becomes slow and induces reverse process of damaging the bone marrow – bones and blood – which in turn slows down the process of creating enough red cells and enough antibodies. Thus the syndrome is weakened and when overworked endocrine glands stop producing vital hormones, this syndrome breaks and the body becomes prone to serious diseases.

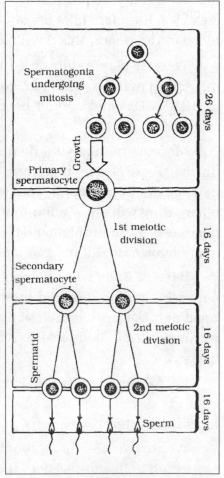

Fig. 34 : Reproduction a sperm

Another cause of 'AIDS' (Acquired Immune Deficiency Syndrome) is sexual relations with persons suffering from 'HIV/AIDS'.

'AIDS' may also be caused through blood transfusion. If blood of person suffering from 'AIDS' is given to a patient, the latter may acquire 'AIDS'. If all the blood collecting agencies, therefore take precaution and care in checking the blood of the donor, this possibility can be prevented.

Thus, it may be observed that self-conscious and self-respecting persons, need not worry about and get frightened of 'HIV AIDS' and should be careful only in taking blood transfusion.

Moreover, if the vital fluid semen is properly preserved till marriage at the right age and not abused (which is possible if the husband and wife remain faithful to each other), they will enjoy a life-time of blissful sex and conjugal happiness. (The problem of HIV/AIDS is discussed in detail in my book "Health in Your Hands : Volume 2".)

**Base of Body :** The human body has an acido-alkaline base which is represented by grey and white matter in the brain and because of their action and reaction, electricity is produced in the body just like electricity produced in a dry battery.

**Recharging of this Life Battery :** Our body has a special built-in device to recharge this inner nonchargeable transistor battery.

When we breathe through the right nostril (as it is connected with sun-positive) the degree of our internal heat increases. In the same way, when we breathe through the left nostril (which is connected with moon-negative) the degree of our internal heat decreases. It has been found recently that the difference between the highest and the lowest temperature is. 09° C. (British Medical Journal)

When we breathe through our right nostril, the air goes into the brain and recharges +ve(Positive) part of our brain cells, grey or white matter (according to Indian Yogic philosophy). At that time, blood recharged with the air breathed in through the right nostril goes into the first ventricle and heat (+ve) is stored. When it reaches the peak level, the current flows towards –ve (negative) and breathing automatically changes to the left nostril. The cooler air then goes in the brain and charges the negative substance, the grey matter (according to Indian yogic philosophy). It is not known whether the white matter represents the (+ve) positive and grey matter represents negative . (–ve) or vice-versa. The blood charged with the air breathed through the left nostril goes into second ventricle and recharges negative till it reaches a peak level and the current flows from the negative to positive. Then, the breathing changes through the right nostril. Thus the change in levels of positive and negative goes on and the electricity so produced goes on flowing into the body. This is why there is an automatic change in the breathing from the right nostril to the left and vice-versa.

Now, when the cerebrospinal fluid passes through the spinal cord and goes down from the brain to the coccyx, because of grey and white matter in the vertebrae, electricity is produced and stored in the prostate where it remains idle called Kundalini – (serpent energy in yoga). Through certain yogic exercises, this latent electric power can be awakened and made to move upwards through different chakras (endocrine glands) *(See fig. 55)*. When it goes up and penetrates through Mooladhar Chakra – (sex glands), the sex power increases. When it penetrates Swadisthan Chakra – (Pancreas – Adrenal), it improves digestion. When it penetrates Vishudha Chakra – (Thyroid – Parathyroid) – it intensifies the process of purifying the body and tends to make it strong. When it penetrates Ajna Chakra – (Pituitary gland) one is able to command and when it penetrates Sahastrar Chakra – (Pineal gland), there is a light which can be seen in the middle of the forehead with closed eyes. In pranic healing, this is called getting Golden Crown on the head.

When the electricity reaches the brain, it slowly activates one by one 20,000 chips of the computer and a sense of new awakening (knowledge) starts emerging from within. One gets new perception of things, a new meaning of life. This process of reviving the latent electricity from the base of the body is called the awakening of Kundalini (the serpent power).

When the electricity penetrates through the Pituitary and Pineal glands, there is a predominance of these glands which in turn changes the whole character and outlook of a person.

From persons having predominance of Pituitary gland, arise great geniuses, eminent literary men, poets, scientists, philosophers, philanthropists and supermen. Persons with dominant Pineal gland, are worshipped in this world as saints, great men, incarnations of god, gifted with divine power. They taste heavenly bliss of self-realisation. They are an embodiment of great wisdom and tenderness and also have strong will power.

The brain cells are so protected that efforts, so far made, in the U. S. A. to recharge them directly have not become successful. However, it is observed, that water charged with gold/silver/copper has a pep-up effect on the assimilation process in our body, as it activates the function of digestion, heart, lungs and creation of cerebrospinal fluid.

That is why in all types of chronic diseases like Cancer, T. B., Asthma, Arthritis, Paralysis, etc., when vitality of the body is at the lowest and in all types of problems of brain, concentrated gold/silver/copper charged water has been found very effective. If at least one glass reduced from two glasses of gold/silver/copper charged water, is taken daily from the age of 50, it could help stop the process of ageing while a proper flow of electricity could be maintained through Acupressure treatment.

**Working of Electricity :** The electricity so produced flows to the brain and re-activates 2.4 to 3.3 billion cells of the brain. These cells are thinner than a hair and stand in a line like the teeth of a comb; when electricity passes the upper part of a cell, it bends and touches the next cell and passes the flow of electricity. When this flow of electric current becomes weak and the flow is otherwise disturbed, the cell dries up and becomes brainsand. Increase in brainsand weakens the flow of electricity – slows down, in turn, the function of the other organs of the body and the ageing process starts. To prevent this process, the brain cells should be recharged; which is possible through gold/silver/copper charged water.

**Flow of Electricity**

Normal                               In old age

Positive + Chi —— Electricity of Body —— Chen — negative

| Earth | Water | Fire | Air | Space |
|---|---|---|---|---|
| Centre is physical structure of body bones, flesh. | Centre is kidney, male & female reproductive organs i.e. testes ovary, lymphatic glands, produce antibodies, sex gland, nerves, tissues, cells, flesh–bone marrow–grow out of semen or the vital fluid ensures fine health. | Centre is stomach spleen, liver, pancreas adrenal produces fire juice i. e., digestive fluid, bile enzymes, maintains body temperature, keeps all the organs active helps formation of blood, flesh, fats, bones. | Centre is chest, lungs heart, thymus, cells forming–main protective-operative of body force, self control-balances, temperament, purity of mind and heart. | Covers entire body, eliminates poison from the body-keeps it healthy & strong, controls thyroid parathyroid tonsils, saliva. nourishes mental nerves and body, induces affection, love unselfish-ness, pre-dominant qualities in females, Pituitary-regulations, sight, hearing discrimination and memory rectify all faults, failings and weakness of five elements and glands Pineal : Controls cerebro spinal fluid, nervous system wisdom, tenderness controls premature Death, Brain–1 generator of electricity (Computer of body). |

Electricity thus controls 2.4 (according to Western philosophy) to 3.3 (according to Indian philosophy) billion brain cells which are found to be of five types representing the five basic main elements of earth, metal, water, fire, air and space. These five elements form the metabolism of our body which controls all the functions as shown in the chart on Page No. 50.

All these five elements and seven endocrine glands are controlled by the electricity of the body.

The same principle of five basic elements is accepted by Acupuncture and is shown in the two figures given below :

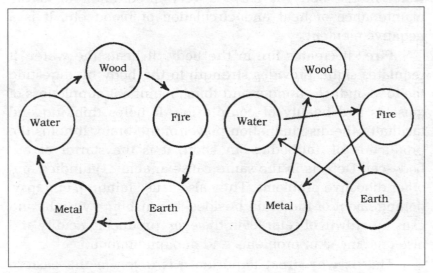

Fig. 35 (a) : Productive cycle        Fig 3.5 (b) : Controlling cycle

The first figure shows the element that helps the other element. While in the second figure, it is shown which element controls the other element and how all these elements are counterbalanced (controlled). Basically, all these elements should remain in proper proportion which is called the Metabolism of the body. **Any disturbance (excess or less) of one element leads to disturbance in other elements and becomes the root cause of a disease.**

**Five Elements :**

**Earth :** All the life forces become inert and inactive in this element and more energy is used to keep it active. People with more weight, flesh, fat, etc. are good example of the predominance of this earth matter in our body. They do not show anxiety, are not eager to acquire any thing. They try to keep away from conflict and their life moves slowly. When there is a disorder of this element in the body, people become selfish and get attached to selfish enjoyments. It is a neutral element.

**Water :** It keeps the flow of body and life. But it has a natural tendency to cool down. As there is more than 70 % water in the body, it plays a very important role in the maintenance of heat and circulation of blood etc. It is a negative element.

**Fire :** It creates fire in the body. It heats the water. It regulates sight, provides strength to the body by digesting the food, induces hunger and thirst, maintains suppleness of muscles and beauty of complexion. It helps thinking and facilitates the discrimination power of the brain. It helps the production of antibodies. In short, it is the starter of our body-car. Defects in the same cause anaemia, jaundice and other digestive problems. They also cause fainting, epilepsy, derangement of the brain besides diminishing eyesight and causing growth of cataract in the eyes, producing acidity and also creating skin problems and depigmentation.

That is why great importance is given in the eastern therapies to control and preserve the element of fire. It is a positive element.

**Air :** Air is life itself. It is the strength and conducts every part of our body. It regulates the function of the heart, circulation of blood and maintains balance of the body. It helps respiration and downward movement of stools and urine. It produces sound, nourishes mental faculties and also the faculty of memory. It moves bile and phlegm (कफ) which cannot move in the body by themselves. It is a positive element.

**Space :** In order that air circulates in the body and maintains a proper balance, there has to be space. If such circulation is blocked, it creates pain even leading to heart attack, paralysis, fainting, etc. It is a negative element.

**Prakruti – Type – different combinations of elements in the body :** If these five basic elements are maintained in proper proportion in the body, a proper metabolism is ensured and the body remains healthy. However, due to heredity, eating and living habits more often than not, we disturb one or two of these elements and thus, upset the metabolism and there is a predominance of three different types of combinations. Such combinations of these elements decide our types – (prakrutis.) Ayurved, the Indian medical therapy, has divided people into three types – (1) Combination through excess of earth + water "(कफ प्रकृति)" (2) Combination through excess of fire + air "(पित्त प्रकृति)" and (3) excess of air element. "(वायु प्रकृति)". This therapy advocates that while treating the patients, one must keep in mind their respective types. For those people having 'kapha prakruti', milk will only create problems. People, therefore, having bronchitis or asthma or indigestion should avoid milk. For people with 'pitt prakruti', spicy food will enhance their problem. Therefore, what is good for one type could be harmful to another.

**Kapha Prakruti :** This is a combination of earth and water. These elements occupy the major portion of our body. Sweet foods and drinks when properly digested are reduced to saline and the blood becomes alkaline. It sustains the body system, increases vigour and there is a marked growth of happiness. It lubricates the joints of bones and keep them working properly. However, this is possible when there is proper element of fire – (heat in the body).

However, because of lack of exercise, overeating, eating between the meals when not hungry, eating more undigestible foods like concentrated sweets, fried things, etc.

cause problems of indigestion and fail to produce enough heat in the body. This, in turn, leads to increase in water content and reduction of heat in the body, resulting in problems like dullness, heaviness, increase in fats, common cold, bronchitis and later on asthma, arthritis, rheumatism, etc.

The best way to cure the above ailments of kapha prakruti is to reduce the intake of undesirable foods, cold drinks and cold foods which only aggravate the problems. These people should eat only light digestble food when hungry, avoid sleeping during the day and over indulgence in sex. Even milk is harmful to them. They should take physical exercises and do more of sun Pranayam.

**Pitta Prakruti :** It is a combination of Fire + Air excess of heat damages the working of brain. It leads to acidity, ulcer, cold due to heat, skin problems, even sex weakness,short temper and falling of hair. Now, in modern times more anxiety, worries, eating more of fried and spicy foods, more exposure to sun, excessive use of antibiotics by people increase their problems. It is, therefore, essential to avoid these things as much as possible.

They should control (1) Adrenal and Pancreas (2) take light purgative of Harde powder ''(हरीतकी चुर्ण)'' with a little sugar for 10 to 12 days in the beginning and then once/twice a week. (3) take sweet fruit juices, first thing in the morning (4) have more fruits, sweet desserts after eating and drink more green juices (5) and do more moon pranayam.

**Air/Vayu Prakruti :** This condition prevails when there is an excess of the element of air. People belonging to this category are more talkative and have day dreams, and are prone to excess sleep and more gas trouble. These imbalances lead to fainting. The tendency to eat heavy-oily foods like fried and foods made out of gram, etc. increases this tendency. People in such condition should avoid constipation and sleeping during day time, have more physical exercise so as to increase heat and circulation and should avoid unsuitable foods. They should do more pranayam.

**Easy way to find out which Prakruti is predominant :**

From $\frac{1}{4}$ glass of water (at room temperature) take one sip; pause; take another sip. And think about the the taste.

| | |
|---|---|
| If it tastes bitter, | it denotes Pitta Prakruti. |
| If it tastes sweet, | it denotes Kapha Prakruti. |
| If it tastes sour, | it denotes Vayu Prakruti. |

Everyone should try and find out the category and type he or she belongs to and avoid as far as possible those items which will aggravate their problems. They should consume food which will suit their type. This is possible with the method shown on page 120 (fig. 68) of this book.

It may be noted that each person is different from the other. So are their tendencies and problems of health. But with proper changes in the diet, good health can be maintained. The cerebro spinal fluid is produced from the blood and so imblance in blood of these basic elements leads to imbalance even in cerebro spinal fluid. More salt in food for instance increases the sodium chloride in cerebro spinal fluid which leads to high B. P. .

Moreover, the climate also plays an important role in its effect on the body. In summer and hot climate, for instance, buttermilk will be useful, but not in monsoon. Therefore, in monsoon buttermilk should be warmed and black pepper and ginger should be added to it before drinking.

Nature grows the required vegetables and fruits etc. suitable for the nourishment of the body in all different areas and seasons. So, wherever possible locally produced seasonal fruits and vegetables should be eaten. Tea grows in parts of Assam and Nilgiris which receive abundant rainfall. Tea is therefore useful in moist climate.

Moreover nature also produces several varieties c´ fruits resembling the shapes of the organs of our body and if eaten regularly they are useful – beneficial to that organ.

| Walnut | = Brain | Mango-Papaya | = Stomach |
|--------|---------|--------------|-----------|
| Almonds | = Eyes | Pears | |
| Apple | = Heart | Guava, | |
| Grapes | = Lungs | and similar | = Ovary |
| | | shaped fruits | |
| Cashewnuts | = Kidney | Banana | = Sex power |
| Kidneybeans | | (Ripe : having black skin) | |

People belonging to one type or the other type of Prakruti can easily find out and eat foods which would do them good and reject foods that will aggravate their problem. It is possible that people have prominence of two types of Prakruti i. e. more of earth + air – which leads to severe gastric trouble or having more of Fire + Air – which leads to ulcers – hot temper etc. In case of serious problems, more than two types of Prakrutis are disturbed-known in Ayurved as Dvidosh (द्विदोष). But in case of very serious problems, like Cancer, all the three types of Prakrutis are found to be disturbed – called Tridosh (त्रिदोष). In such cases it is utmost necessary to take proper care of diet and balancing the effects of medicines on tendencies.

This practice will also enable us to prevent wasting our energy in digesting and expelling these food intakes not suitable to our body.

**Energy :** In order that the body and brain can function properly, it is necessary to create energy from the five basic elements. That is why we take food and drinks.

The whole cosmos gets its energy from the sun. All types of natural foods, fruits, vegetables, cereals, pulses, etc. have in them almost equal measure of positive and negative of sun energy. However, foods contain positive and negative properties in varying degrees. All foods can be divided in six tastes which all foods/drinks have :

| | | | |
|---|---|---|---|
| Bitter | = Air + Space | Sweet | = Earth + Water |
| Astringent | = Air + Water | Salty | = Earth + Fire |
| Pungent (hot) | = Air + Fire | Sour | = Water + Fire |

*(as per Charak Samhita)*

In our daily diet it is necessary to maintain a proper balance of all these six tastes. Surprisingly, Ayurved, the Indian medical science, has made elaborate research in all kinds of fruits, vegetables and minerals and has established their after effects on the human system. Medical students should study this dietary system with great care.

By taking foods more of negative types or more of positive types, we create imbalances, leading to diseases. The body tries to balance that positive and negative excesses in the system and its efforts are called disease. In Acupuncture, the expert tries to bring this balance between positive (chi +) and negative (chen –).

Surprisingly, China has made indepth research in energy derived from food and has come to the conclusion that one's food intake should consist of 65 % in cereals and pulses like wheat-rice-millets, grams, etc. and the balance 35 % in milk-milk products, vegetables, dry fruits, oils, etc. these would be the ideal contents of a balanced diet.

After the body is fully developed one must eat and drink only those things which are suitable to one's body (see page 120) and only when one feels hungry. The fruits and vegetables have in them a natural storage of the sun's energy and if we make a daily practice of having one glass of fruit juice and two to three cups of green juice of vegetables, our requirement for food will be reduced to a minimum and we will have enough energy to maintain the body in a healthy condition. This change in diet has been successfully tried in cases of chronic diseases including cancer and results are astounding. Deficiency of nutrition can be greatly reduced by green juice. (page 169)

Such a practice on a mass scale will lead to less requirement of food and help **prevent wastage of food and famine conditions.**

**Working of Atomic Reactor-i. e. Production of Energy :** Chemicals, which are created from the food we eat, through a chemical process and oxygen are supplied to the brain by blood. This is like petrol in a car. The quadruplicate cells in the brain generate constant sparks in it and through a combustion there, energy H+ (Hydrogen) is produced which in turn creates the necessary heat and energy. Excess of this heat is thrown out of the body through exhalation. However, if there remains excess of it, it creates problems and to remove the same, through electric process the body turns it into $H_2O$ to be thrown out as common cold.

**Control of Body :**
**Through Nucleic Acids :** The picture below is that of a brain cell. The nucleus of a cell contains nearly all its DNA and 10 % of its RNA. Both nucleic acids are involved in directing the primary synthesis of protein molecules that in turn act as structural elements (enzymes or hormones) as under :

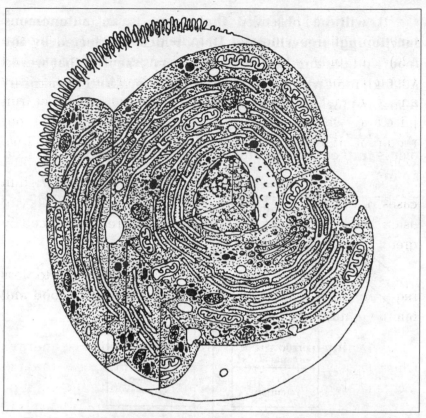

Fig. 36 : Brain Cell as seen in a Three-Dimensional Electron micrograph

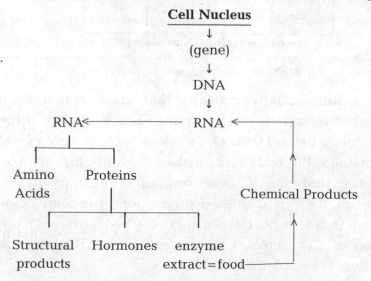

It will be observed that there is an autonomous functioning – (recycling) of DNA which is effected by the food we take and therefore, it is very essential that we do not take food which will aggravate our prakruti (weakness-tendency) for any particular basic element.

**PH Level and Death :** The necessity to have a balanced diet is further corroborated by a close look at the following figure.

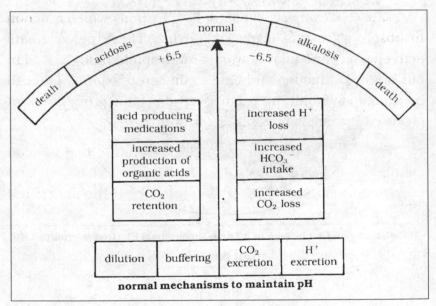

Fig. 37 : Normal mechanisms to maintain pH

This figure clearly indicates that there should be a balance between positive acids and negative alkalies in the body within a normal level of +6.5 and −6.5. If such a level is maintained, the body remains healthy and efficient. You will notice that due to over-working of acid producing mechanism, there is increased production of organic acids and when these are not thrown out of the body, there is more retention of $CO_2$ (creates excess heat). This disturbs the power flow of electricity in the body.

In the same way, when there is an increased loss of heat due to continuous cold (when more water $H_2O$ is thrown out of our system) there is an excess of alkalies in the body leading to degeneration.

The level of positive and negative bioelectricity is called PH. This level should remain between $+6.5$ PH and $-6.5$ PH. If due to any reason this PH level is not maintained, death takes place.

This PH level is well maintained by pons which function to absorb excess of acids and toxins. These pons remain active with the regular flow of cerebro spinal fluid created in our brain. Production and balance in cerebrospinal fluid can be maintained only by a balanced diet and proper flow of electricity which is possible by Acupressure.

For every living being Death is definite, but we can maintain our body, remain healthy till our last breath and here Acupressure can play a vital role as it is the only 'Do it yourself therapy' which teaches us how to send the life current to all parts of the body, how to control all endocrine glands. It is the ONLY THERAPY, which gives Prevention, proper Diagnosis without Tests and costs and yet equal to such Diagnosis made with MRI test; and surprisingly CURE for all types of A to Z diseases. According to Acupressure, all types of cancer are the easiest diseases to be cured. It may be noted that HEALTH IS OUR BIRTHRIGHT and we can easily achieve it.

———

# CHAPTER 3

# ACUPRESSURE : THERAPY AND PRACTICE

From the study of these first two chapters you must have come to know that the greatest wonder in this cosmos is the human body. Our body is well equipped with the best, automatic, delicate but the most powerful machines – Heart and Lungs (a non-stop pumping set); Eyes – a wonderful camera-cum-projector system; Ears – an astounding sound system; Stomach – a wonderful chemical laboratory; Nerves – miles of communication system. Brain – an unparalleled computer with infinite capacity. And the greatest thing about it is the unbelievable co-ordination of all these machines so that this body can easily work for over a hundred years or more.

It is a fact that in any good machine, provision is made whereby it automatically stops when there is a danger and restarts when you push its switch e. g. refrigerator and hot water geyser. It is not surprising that such a provision is made in the human body also. It is true that the system of our body is very intricate. But to maintain it is easy. Nature has provided in our body an 'in-built mechanism' to maintain these machines and to repair them if need be. This science of health which makes use of this in-built mechanism is popularly known as Acupressure. This therapy is the most precious gift to mankind from the Creator Himself.

The Acupressure therapy was known in India even 5000 years ago, (according to Sushrut Samhita). Unfortunately, it was not preserved properly and went to Sri Lanka (Ceylon) in the form of Acupuncture. From Sri Lanka (Ceylon), this therapy was taken to China and Japan by Buddhist monks or nomadic Aryans took it there and at present China is teaching Acupuncture to the world. This therapy was known to the Red Indians way back in the sixteenth century. In the twentieth century, researches have been made in the U.S.A. which have contributed greatly to the development of this therapy. It is practised by many Allopathic and Naturopathic doctors there. Now, the World Health Organization, too, has paid attention to this simple and easy therapy.

The word 'Acupressure' is related to 'Acupuncture'. 'Acu' means a needle and 'puncture' means to 'pierce'. Acupuncture means the art of treating diseases by piercing specific points in the body. Acupressure means the art of treating diseases by applying pressure on specific points with the help of one's thumb or unpointed things.

**Principle :** As mentioned in Chapter 2 our body consists of five basic elements :

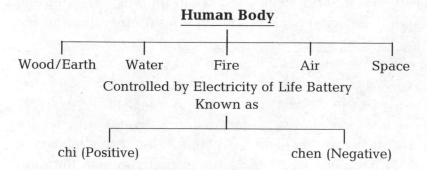

**Human Body**

| Wood/Earth | Water | Fire | Air | Space |

Controlled by Electricity of Life Battery
Known as

chi (Positive)                    chen (Negative)

These five elements are controlled by the electricity of the body known in the West as Bio-Electricity. The current of electricity, 'Chetana', comes from this non-changeable Life Battery. This battery has been installed in our body at the time of conception. The white dazzling light generated by this battery can be seen in the middle of one's forehead with eyes closed, through certain Yogic methods. Many people, including myself, have seen this light.

Out of this battery, electric current ('चेतना') passes in the body through the lines shown in fig. 38. These lines known as 'Meridians' start from the tip of each finger of the right hand, go all over the body and end in the toes of the right foot and so also on the left side. Now so long as this current of electricity flows properly in the body, the body remains fit and healthy. If for any reason this current does not reach any part of the body, there is malfunctioning of that part accompained by pain in some cases, if not attended to in time, it may invite illness. So, if the current is properly sent to the affected parts, the pain, if any, would subside and the disease of malfunctioning of that part would be cured. Thus, Acupressure is the Science of Nature which teaches us to cure diseases through the in-built mechanism of the body – the technique of how to send the current to all the desired parts of the body.

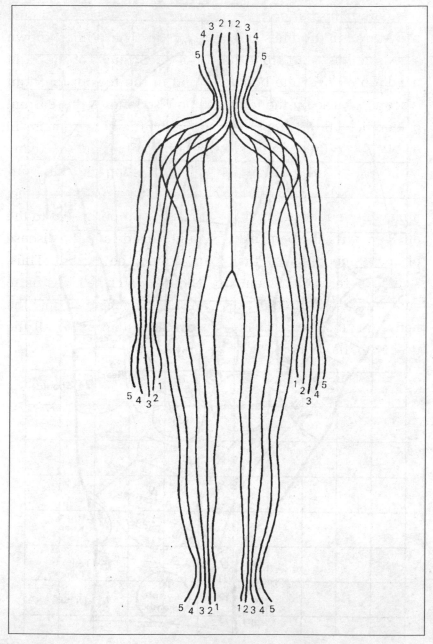

Fig. 38
Flow of *(Chetana)* electric current-lines
(meridians) which are divided into
5 zones each on the right and left sides.

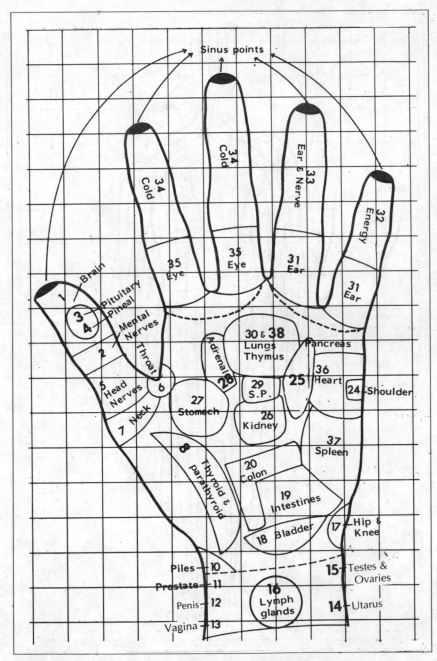

**Fig. 39 (a) : Left-Hand**
Location and Number of points connected
with different organs and endocrine glands.

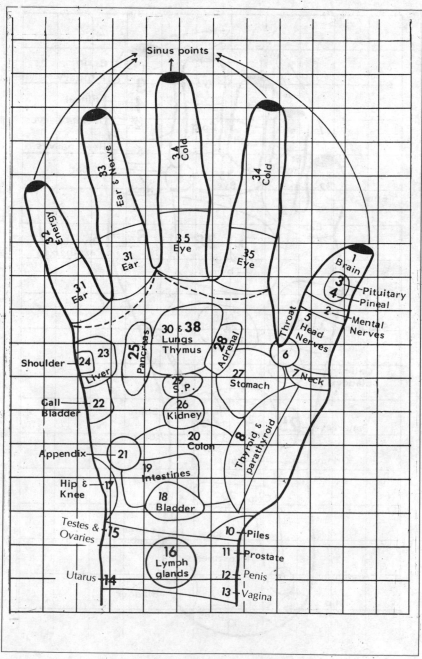

Fig. 39 (b) : Right-Hand
For treatment : Pressure is to be applied
on and around these points of palms

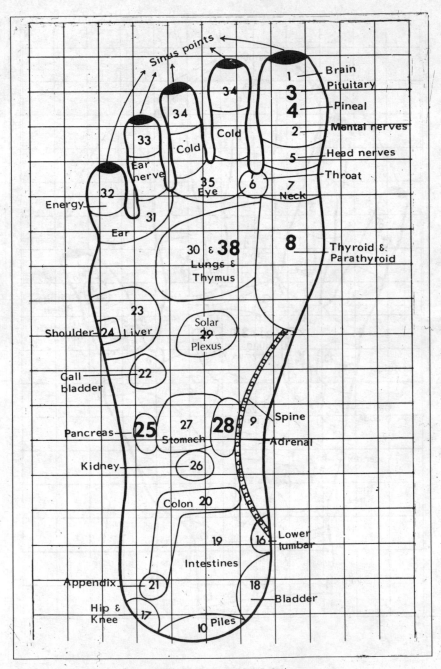

**Fig. 40 (a) : Right-Sole**
For treatment : Pressure is to be applied
on and around these points of the soles

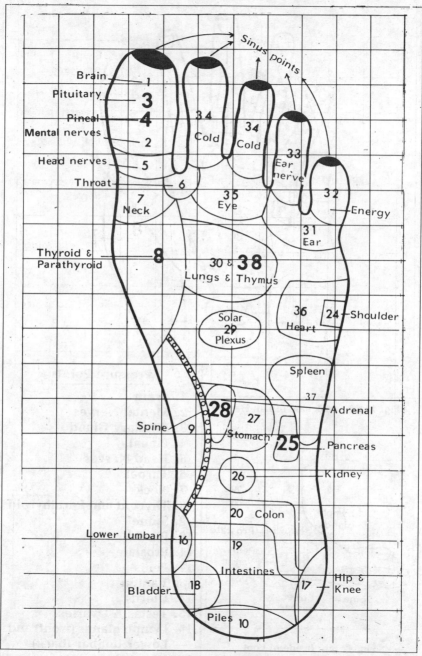

**Fig. 40 (b) : Left-leg Sole**
Location and Number of points connected
with different organs and endocrine glands

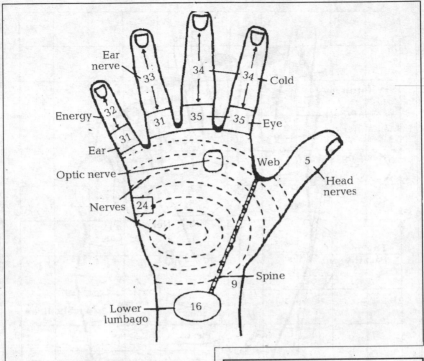

Fig. 41 (a) : Back side of Left Hand

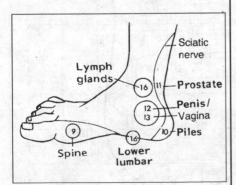

Fig. 42 (a) : Inside of Foot

## Pressure Points

1. **Brain**
2. **Mental Nerves**
3. **Pituitary Gland**
4. **Pineal**
5. **Head Nerves**
6. **Throat**
7. **Neck**
8. **Thyroid and Parathyroid**
9. **Spine**
10. **Piles**
11. **Prostate**
12. **Penis**
13. **Vagina**
14. **Uterus**
15. **Testes & Ovaries**
16. **Lymph glands (front) and Lower lumbar (back)**
17. **Hip and Knee**
18. **Bladder**
19. **Intestines**

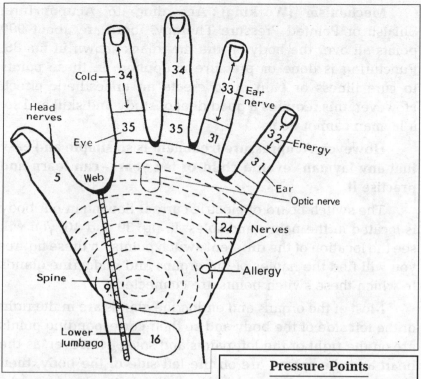

**Fig. 41 (b) : Back side of Right Hand**

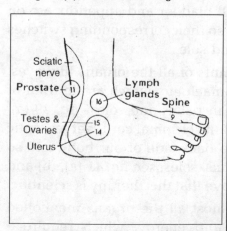

**Fig. 42 (a) : Outside of Foot**

| Pressure Points |
| --- |
| 20. Colon |
| 21. Appendix (front) |
|     Allergy (back side) |
| 22. Gall Bladder |
| 23. Liver |
| 24. Shoulder |
| 25. Pancreas |
| 26. Kidney |
| 27. Stomach |
| 28. Adrenal |
| 29. Solar Plexus |
| 30. Lungs |
| 31. Ear |
| 32. Energy |
| 33. Nerves of Ear |
| 34. Cold |
| 35. Eyes |
| 36. Heart |
| 37. Spleen |
| 38. Thymus |

**Mechanism (Working) :** According to Acupuncture, Shiatsu or Pointed Pressure Therapy, there are about 900 points all over the body on the meridians shown in fig. 38. Puncturing is done or pressure is applied on these points to cure illness or pain or to create an anaesthetic effect. However, this requires a good deal of study and skill and so, a layman cannot do it.

**However, Acupressure treatment is so simple and easy that any layman – even a child of ten years – can learn and practise it.**

The switch board of electric current flowing in our body is located in the palms and soles. In fig. 39 and 40, you will see the location of the different switch points. In these figures you will find the names of the organs and endocrine glands to which these switch points are connected.

Most of the organs and endocrine glands are in the right or the left side of the body and so their corresponding points are on the right or the left palms and soles. However, as the heart and the spleen are on the left side of the body, their corresponding points are only on the left palm and sole. Similarly, since, the liver, gall bladder and appendix are on the right side of the body and so their corresponding switches are only on the right palm and sole.

In the same way, the points of all the organs like eyes, throat, ears, heart, lungs, stomach etc. which are in front of the body are shown in front in palms and soles – fig. 39 (a), (b) and 40 (a), (b). And the points of spinal cord, nerves, optic nerve, allergy etc. are on the back side of our body and so are shown on the back of palms/soles. see fig. 41 (a), (b) and 42 (a), (b). These divisions prove that this therapy is scientific.

We are familiar with almost all the organs mentioned above except Solar Plexus and energy, which require a special mention and hence are explained in detail below :

**Solar Plexus (Point No. 29) :** This is also known as 'Nabhi Chakra' – ('नाभिचक्र') the controlling centre for all the organs below the diaphragm. This concept of *'Nabhi Chakra'* is not found in any other therapies except in 'Ayurved', the Indian Medical Science of Life. This proves that this therapy had originated in India. For disturbances in all the organs below the diaphragm it is necessary to apply pressure treatment to this Point No. 29.

**Methods to confirm whether the Solar Plexus is in order or not :**

( 1 ) In the morning, on an empty stomach, when you lie down on a flat surface on your back and if you press your finger or thumb in the navel, you will feel a throbbing sound just like that of the heart. That means the system is O.K.

If this throbbing is found anywhere above the navel, it means that Solar Plexus has shifted upwards. Sameway, if such throbbing is found anywhere below navel, it means that Solar Plexus has shifted downwards. And so it is necessary to correct the same by any methods mentioned below.

( 2 ) Lie down on your back. Keep the arms (hands) straight on your sides. Keep legs straight and the toes upright. The two big toes should be in level, if they are not, it indicates disturbance in the Solar Plexus.

( 3 ) Join the two palms as per fig (a) shown here and match the lines of No. 1 (i. e. heart lines as per Astrology). At that time, if the Solar Plexus is in order, the upper line in small finger No. 4 shown in figure will match. If the Solar Plexus has shifted, the line No. 4 will not match.

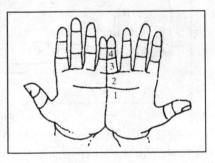

Figure (a)

This centre shifts upward or downward when excess weight is lifted or when there is severe gas trouble. In such cases, the throbbing will not be noticed in the centre of the navel, but it will be noticed somewhere around the navel. The upward shifting of the Solar Plexus leads to constipation and downward shifting brings more motions every time when there is a pressure. This cannot be cured by drugs. And when these problems persist, it can damage the digestive system and may require an operation. It may even lead to Cancer. One of the causes of Cancer of Colon (lower, and greater part of the large intestine) is chronic constipation. In such cases, it has been found that this Solar Plexus has moved upwards. It is, therefore, advisable to check the position of Solar Plexus before starting any treatment. The Solar Plexus is like the mainspring of a watch. Unless it is set right, treatment may not give the desired results.

**Methods to bring the Solar Plexus to order :** These are to be done only on an empty stomach in the morning or 3 to 4 hours after meals.

( 1 ) By pushing the throbbing towards the centre of the navel.

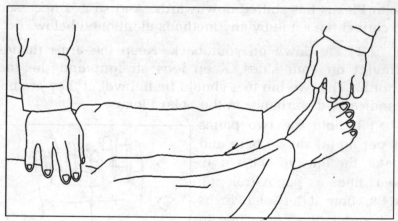

**Fig. 43**

( 2 ) By putting weight on the navel and trying to press it towards the centre.

( 3 ) Ask the patient to lie down on the back on a flat surface and keep the arms straight on the sides. Then with one hand apply pressure on the knee of the leg of which the big toe is at a lower level and with other hand keeping the long finger between two big toes, try to pull up the big toe which is lower. Repeat this action 2 to 4 times till both the big toes come in level (refer fig. 43).

( 4 ) By putting up a small oil lamp/candle on the navel (a coin or something can be kept on the navel as a base to

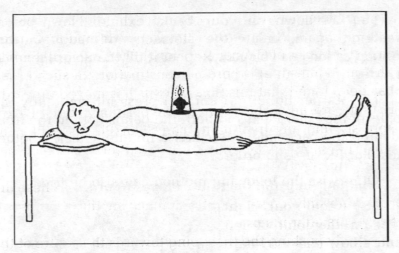

**Fig. 44**

hold the candle), cover it with a metal glass and press it for a minute (as shown in figure 44). The air inside will burn out and a vacuum will be created. This vacuum will bring the Solar Plexus to the centre. Then lift the glass from one side after one minute. Repeat this three to four times till the throbbing is felt at the centre.

(5) Lie down on your back, keep the arms on the sides and the head on the ground without pillow. Lift both the legs and bring them up to 90° from the ground as shown in the figure. After this, bring the

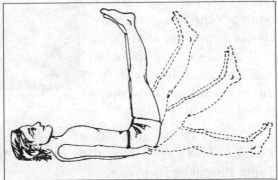

**Fig. 45**

legs as slowly as possible on the ground keeping them straight and without lifting the head from the ground. Repeat the same five to six times and feel the throbbing *(See fig. 45)*.

(6) Lie down on your back, exhale. Now, before breathing again, inflate the stomach and maintain that position as long as you can. Repeat it till the Solar Plexus is in order.

(7) As per fig. 39 (a) and (b) press intermittently the points of the Solar Plexus in both the palms both in the front side and the back side. After half a minute, check whether the Solar Plexus is in order.

Otherwise the following method can also be tried.

(8) Keep your right palm on the joint of left hand elbow and hold hard the muscles there. Then with a jerk bring up the left hand and try to touch the left shoulder with the open thumb. Repeat five times. In the same way, do it on the right hand five times. Then check if the Solar Plexus is in order as per fig. (a) on page 73. This is one of the easiest way. Hence, you are advised to do so every morning without worrying whether the Solar Plexus is in order or not.

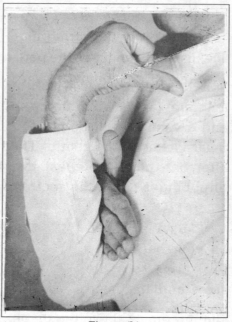

Figure (b)

This can be done every day morning on an empty stomach or 3 to 4 hours after meals. **Please ensure that the Solar Plexus is in order.**

After correcting the Solar Plexus, drink water or milk adding dry ginger in it.

**What to do in case of frequent shifting of the Solar Plexus :** Due to severe gas trouble, **weakness of intestines,** lifting of **heavy articles,** sometimes, there is frequent shifting of Solar Plexus. In such cases, it gets shifted in the afternoon even though, it was corrected in the morning. Do the following :

First correct the Solar plexus. Take a little string (thicker than the sewing thread) and tie eight to nine rounds of this thread around the base of big toe and tie a knot. Do the same with the other big toe. (It should not be very tight). Ask the patient to keep it on for a minimum of three days. The Solar Plexus will remain in order.

During this period if there is unbearable pain in the big toes, then only this string may be removed. Once the Solar Plexus has been fixed, the patient can check it every alternate day and correct it if necessary. For complete cure, the patient must have a diet of green juices, fruit juices and light food. The patient should also do some exercises to strengthen the muscles of digestive organs. Also check up about worms and remove them, if necessary, by the method shown later on in chapter 14. Since the Solar Plexus is like mainspring/quartz of a watch, it must always be kept in order.

Whenever the complaint about constipation or loose motions continues, first check up the Solar Plexus and correct it, if necessary.

Similarly, for any problem of any organ below the diaphragm or above the diaphragm like heart, please check up the Solar Plexus and correct it. e.g. pain in abdomen, stomach, etc. or pain in chest/heart or even in case the medical adviser informs that the heart is enlarged.

**Case study :** (a) "A patient was getting pain in chest quite often. Every time. E.C.G. would be taken. But it would be normal. X'Ray showed enlarged heart. The Solar Plexus was corrected. Pain stopped and next X'Ray confirmed that heart was normal."

(b) A patient was suffering from Hiatus Hernia. He was advised operation. His Solar Plexus was corrected; within 2 days, his trouble disappeared.

(c) A lady Doctor, a gynaecologist, was suffering from pain in abdomen for many years. Her Solar Plexus was corrected and then she became alright.

(d) A young girl, could not retain any food or even drink. She would vomit it out. She was kept in a leading hospital in Mumbai for 21 days. No diagnosis was made. The complaint continued and developed into acute colic pains; at that time she would toss from side to side on a double bed. The root cause was found in the disturbance of the Solar Plexus.It was corrected, she stopped vomitting. She was put on green juices and fruit juices. Within a week, she became normal.

(e) A patient was advised operation of colon-because of long term problem of fistula. Only 3 days before the date of the operation, he consulted an Acupressurist. His Solar Plexus was corrected. And recovery was so fast that operation was not found necessary.

**Energy (Point No. 32) :** When you feel tired or have passed sleepless nights, you will feel pain on the point, which means recharging has not been done properly. It is essential at such a time to give treatment on that point and drink lukewarm water, preferably Health Drink or charged water. *(Details about the Health Drink and charged water are given in chapter 14.)*

**Webs :** Over and above all these points, it is necessary to apply pressure on the webs. The large one is situated between the thumb and the first finger and the small ones are between the fingers. And so also between the toes. These webs are the starting points for the nerves and so pressure should be applied on these points daily *(See fig. 46)*.

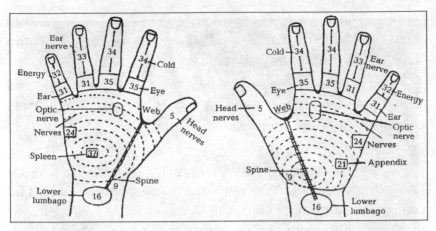

**Fig. 46**

**Method of Pressure :** According to this therapy, pressure is to be applied on and around all points on the two palms and soles only. That will send the current to the corresponding organs and activate them. For example, when you press Point No. 1 shown on the thumb, the current will flow to the brain. When you press deeper on the point of any of the endocrine glands which are called the controllers of all organs, the current is sent there and it corrects the function of that particular gland i.e. if the gland is functioning less efficiently, it will be activated and normalised. However, if it is working more vigorously, it will reduce its activity and bring it to normal. **Thus, simply by appling pressure on the points of the endocrine glands, we are able to control these most vital glands.**

Pressure can be applied by pressing with the thumb or the first finger on the point or with unsharpened pencil etc. *(See fig. 47, 48 & 49)* or by massaging that point and around it. **The pressure is to be applied intermittently like pumping and continued pressure is to be avoided.** This action is to be repeated for 1 to 2 minutes.

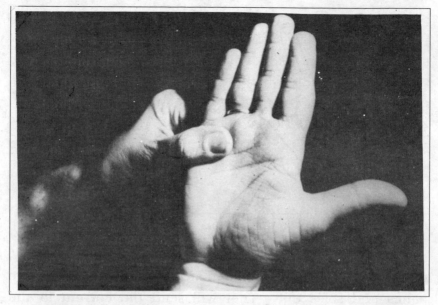

Fig. 47 : Picture showing how to apply pressure with a horizontal thumb

**How much pressure to be applied :** *The pressure to be applied should be just enough for you to be able to feel it.* However, on all the points of the endocrine glands. viz. Point Nos. 3, 4, 8, 14, 15, 16, 25, 28 and 38 shown bold in the figures

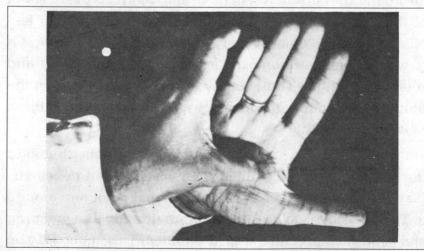

Fig. 48 : Picture showing how to apply deeper pressure on the points of endocrine glands with vertical thumb

which are situated in the middle of the body, deeper pressure is to be applied. This can be done with the verticle thumb as shown in fig. 48 or with an unsharpened pencil or a wooden stick as shown in fig. 49. Except on these points of endocrine glands, pressure is to be applied on all other points by keeping the thumb horizontal.

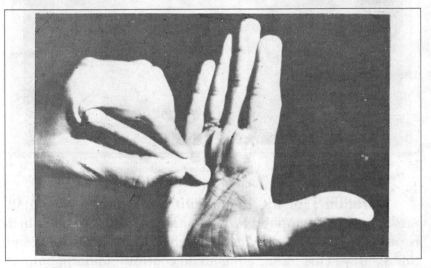

Fig. 49 : Picture showing how to apply deeper pressure on the point of endocrine glands with a blunt or rounded wooden stick

**Body and its subdivisions :** Our body is divided into two parts, the right side and the left side. For anything wrong with the organs or the parts on the right side of the body, treatment is to be given on the corresponding points of the palm of the right hand or the sole of the right foot, and vice versa on the left side.

Further, the body is subdivided into front and back. For the spine, nerves, back, lower lumbago, sciatic nerve and hips, pressure is to be applied on the back of the palms and soles *(See fig. 50)*. But for all other organs and endocrine glands, the pressure is to be applied on the palms or soles. Refer to figs. 39 (a), (b) and 40 (a), (b) on pages 66, 67, 68 and 69.

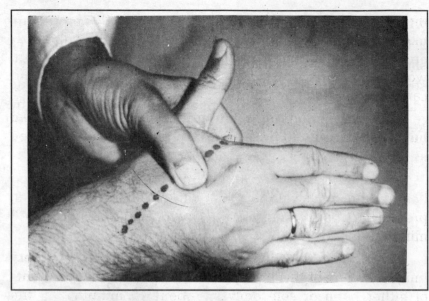

**Fig. 50 : Picture showing how to apply pressure on
the spinal cord (Point No. 9) on the back of the palm**

**Duration :** For the treatment of any disease or organ, pressure is to be applied for one minute on each point which is paining when pressed and this has to be repeated three times a day. This treatment is to be continued till the pain on these points subsides.

**Threefold Benefits of Acupressure :**

( 1 ) PREVENTION of all types of diseases including heart problem, paralysis and even cancer.

( 2 ) Instant and proper DIAGNOSIS without any tests and cost and yet equal to that of MRI test.

( 3 ) CURE of all types of diseases including that of cancer/brain and even HIV/AIDS.

**( 1 ) How to maintain good health :** You will observe that all the points on the palms are up to 1 inch below the wrist. So, without bothering about where the different points are situated, you should start pressing from one inch from the wrist i.e. Point No. 16 and slowly press the full palm and all the fingers on both the front and back side. By pressing both the palms or soles for five minutes each, you will cover all the points thus stimulating all the organs of the body. It is like complete servicing of the car. And when all the organs are properly stimulated and the endocrine glands are working properly, you will feel more agile and energetic and can maintain good health.

**Remember that continuous pressure is not to be applied but only intermittent pressure like pumping is to be applied as mentioned above.**

**For children under 5 :** For maintaining general good health and physical development of children below 5, pressure to be applied on each palm and sole for 2 to 3 minutes.

**Prevention of Sickness or Disease :** This is a very unique feature of this therapy. When you press all the points of either palm or sole daily for about 10 minutes, all the organs are activated and recharged like a battery cell and all the endocrine glands are normalized. The net result of this is that all the organs and glands of the body get properly aligned and they function properly, as a result of which health is maintained and the possibility of any type of disease, including that of cancer, is greatly reduced.

**( 2 ) Wonderful Way of Diagnosis-Medical Check-up :** By taking this treatment (pressing all the points daily for 10 minutes) you not only maintain good health but also get a **FREE MEDICAL CHECK-UP.**

It may so happen that when you pressed all the points yesterday, there was no pain on any point; it means that you were in good health. But today when you press all the points, you may find some pain inside or around some point, that means there is something wrong with the organ connected with that point. And this disturbance has developed in the body during the last 24 hours. Any pain or disease of any organ or part of the body is reflected in the corresponding point of the palms or soles. That is why this therapy is also called 'Reflexology'. When you find the pain, it can be said in the language of electricity that the 'Fuse' has gone from that part. That point would be found tender. So when you press, the part below that point. It hurts. **Thus, you become your own doctor and can diagnose the disease instantly without any cost or laboratory tests.**

It is possible that for the first two days you may not get any response from pressing your points because uptill now you have not used them. However, from the third day, you will start getting the response.

In case there is no pain on the points on palms when pressed, press the same points in the soles. Most probably you will observe pain on the points in the soles.

It is most important for any medical practitioner to have the correct diagnosis of the problem of the patient before proceeding with the treatment. The correct diagnosis is possible only when the root cause is found out. It will be observed that apart from physical checking, it is necessary for the doctors to have urine report, blood report, X'ray, cardiogram, sonography and brain scanning, etc. before the diagnosis is made. That is a lengthy and costly procedure which most of the patients cannot afford.

Because of the rapid scientific progress, the training necessary to master the techniques of diagnosis has become long and expensive. In Ayurvedic, Acupuncture and *Unani* systems, for example, diagnosis can be made by an expert thorough the knowledge of *Nadis* (नाड़ी) and as such its study takes more than six to ten years. In Homeopathy, prolonged sessions with patients are necessary and so very few patients can be attended to even by an experienced Homeopath. While, treatment under Nature Cure is lengthy and there also the Naturopaths in most cases do not go to the root cause. They try to purify the body and leave the work of cure to awakened and enriched *Chetana*.

However, according to Acupressure, the switchboard of this Bio-Electricity is in palms and soles. In the figs. 39 and 40, you will see the various points connected with their respective corresponding organs of the body. It is further observed that so long as this flow of bio-electricity-life current is reaching all the organs properly, there will be NO PAIN on these points when pressed. **You will be surprised to note that acupressure is the only therapy which prevents disease and helps a person to maintain good health.** In order to achieve this, you simply have to press the full palm/sole slowly for 5 minutes and the other palm/sole for 5 minutes and when the patient is over 40 years, for two minutes in the one inch circle in the middle of right forearm (See fig. 81). Thus, by simply pressing both the palms/soles like pumping in ten minutes, you are recharging all the vital organs. It is like servicing or realigning a car. When all the vital organs are working normally, the possibility of a disease becomes very remote. Thus, just by pressing your palms or soles for 5–5 minutes each, every day. you will not only prevent any disease but enjoy good health.

"FREE MEDICAL CHECK-UP. At the same time, you also get a free medical check-up of the complete body.

**Diagnosis :** Owing to overworking of these organs or due to some other cause, when an organ is damaged, carbon dioxide/toxins gather around that organ and when pressed on the connecting point of the organ either in the palm or in the sole of the legs; you will feel pain. **This pain is unpleasant and totally different from the experience of pressure given on that point. And at that time, there will be a flicker, in the eyes of the patient.** So, even without any information from the patient or without any tests the diagnosis can be made just by giving pressure on different points located in palms/soles. It will be interesting for you, to know that I have been challenged on several occasions to diagnose the problems without being given any background or case history of the patient. I will quote in this regard only one incident.

Mr. Narain Dutt Tiwari, former Union Minister of India for finance and former Chief Minister of Uttar Pradesh, called me to his hotel at Santacruz airport. His wife is a qualified

Allopathic Gynaec doctor. She asked me to examine her husband and diagnose his problems. One by one, I pressed the different points of the palms. In 2 minutes I told her about the improper working of five different organs. Then when I told her that her husband was suffering from piles and had long-rooted constipation. She nearly jumped up, duly amazed, I told her that the Solar Plexus of Mr. Tiwari was not in order. He was asked to lie down and it was found that the level of the big two toes was not equal – right big toe was more than one inch higher than the left big toe. It was immediately corrected. Mr Tiwari was asked to give pressure on chin to remove constipation and according to the information received later, within a week his disease of piles was completely cured due to proper diagnosis and correct treatment by Acupressure.

**Thus, you will observe that the pain felt at any point on the palms or soles when pressed is a clear indication of some problem connected with that organ.** The body is divided into right and left parts, so any problem connected with the right side of the body will be reflected on the points on the right palm or sole and vice versa. Further, the points of our body are subdivided into front and back. All the organs situated in the front part of the body e.g. eyes, heart, stomach, etc. are situated on the palms or in soles and the points connected with the organs on the back part are situated at the back of palms or on the upper side of the soles e.g. spinal cord, etc.

It is interesting to note that the diagnosis made this way is so accurate that on several occasions, I had to challenge the diagnosis made with results of the X-rays and Sonography. I shall quote three instances.

( 1 ) An athlete was advised operation of the spinal cord on the basis of few X-rays examinations. He approached me and I told him that as there is no pain on Point No. 9 of the spinal cord, there was no damage to the spinal cord, and so operation was not necessary. And the root cause of his severe back pain was found in the damage to his Sciatic Nerve. He was taught how to take treatment with this 'Do it yourself therapy' and within 10 days he was alright.

(2) A gentleman was suffering from jaundice, according to diagnosis on the basis of X'rays and Sonography; he was told that there was stone-obstruction in his gall bladder and operation was necessary. I was called three days prior to operation. After examining the patient in three minutes; I told him that there is nothing wrong with the gall bladder. Liver was damaged and the stone was near the kidney. His heart was in a sound condition. So if he so desired operation can be done. He was operated upon and his gall bladder was removed and even after a minute bisection, no stone was found. After 4 hours of operation, the patient was put under X'rays. The stone was found near kidney. They continued the operation for 8 hours and the stone was removed. Luckily, the heart condition of the patient was good and so he survived.

(3) A patient was told on the basis of X'rays and examination that he had cancer of the mouth and operation was necessary. When called to the hospital, after not even 2 minutes of examination, I told him that there was no cancer but only soreness in the throat. Doctor insisted on operation only to find that there was no cancer.

**Thus you will observe that without any instruments or costly tests, exact diagnosis is possible with this Nature's Health Science of Acupressure. And this checkup is not only equal to that of MRI Test but instant also.**

When a patient comes to you, the very first thing you can do is to press on Point No. 8 of Thyroid-parathyroid. If there is no pain there, the problem is a minor one, because if there is a continued problem in the body for more than 8/10 days, this point of thyroid is first to be disturbed and when pressed there will be pain. In such a case, you can go on pressing the various other points as per the patient's complaints.

Many a time, it is observed that young men never disclose their sex problems. Similarly ladies in India also feel shy in discussing their problems about menses, sex, etc. Therefore, even by pressing on Point Nos. 11 to 15 of sex glands, these problems can be diagnosed.

Now, I will tell you about the exactness of this diagnosis. I was invited by an eye specialist at his residence. He asked me to examine his 27 year old son. After examining the palms, I told him that there was tonsil on the right side and only reddishness on the left side of throat. Doctor called for a torch and a spoon, examined the throat of his son and **admitted that my diagnosis was perfectly correct.**

The wonderful part of this diagnosis is that the patient can himself find out his problem. One gentleman had pain in the chest. He feared heart attack. Cardiogram was taken in the hospital and as there was no abnormality, he was discharged after 4 days. Later on every time he had pain in chest, he would call for a doctor, get his cardiogram and be satisfied to confirm that it was normal. He was presented with my book. Afterwards whenever he had any chest pain, he would examine his Point No. 36 of heart and would be relieved of anxiety in a minute on feeling no pain on that point. During one year alone he saved over one thousand dollars and had great amount of relief.

You will be surprised to know that the dreaded disease of cancer can be detected only in two minutes. In cancer detection centres or hospitals cancer can be detected only when it has already developed more than 40 %, while with this method it can be detected even when it is hardly 5 %. Moreover, the exact location of cancer can be traced. I was asked by a lady to diagnose her problem. After examining her palms, I was forced to tell her just in two minutes that she had cancer on her right breast. She then admitted having got her right breast operated for cancer. I told her that cancer was not totally cured and it had started affecting the liver.

She started Acupressure treatment, got cured within 6 weeks and even after 6 years, she enjoys good health.

This type of diagnosis is very useful in case of children, as they are not able to tell or explain their problems. Just by pressing on different points on the soles the exact root cause of the disease can be found out, because while you are pressing the soles, the child will cry out or withdraw the sole when any point is paining. Later on, the child can be given this treatment along with bio-chemic medicines.

**Thus, with the help of Acupressure, a perfect diagnosis can be made.** The patient is not expected to know the name of his disease because there are thousands of names for diseases. But all the diseases are connected with the vital organs of the body. And Acupressure can diagnose as to which organ is damaged.

After the diagnosis is made, in the treatment of most of the diseases, the patient can use this therapy and get cured. However, in case of chronic and serious diseases, two or three therapies—Homeopathy, Ayurved, Chromotherapy Natureopathy etc. can be combined to bring faster relief to the patient.

A lady on the basis of X'ray and other tests was put on Dialysis—3 times a week. Later on she was told that both the kidneys have almost failed and she is required to have transplantation of her kidney. It would cost her rupees 3,00,000 or about 8,000 US dollars. She got scared and came to me. Thorough examination was made and in five minutes, I told her that there was a minor trouble in kidneys and she can be cured within 15 days. The root cause of her problem was cancer in the uterus. She was then asked to take treatment at home. Within 15 days all the swellings were gone and she passed clear urine quite frequently. She became energetic and with a further treatment of 30 days, she was cured.

That is why when a patient comes to you, please do not be carried away by what he says. Get your hints from the symptoms narrated to you and just think about the root cause and within a minute you will be able to locate the exact root cause of the trouble.

In case of common cold, tonsilitis, sinusitis, asthma, etc. many times the root cause is cold due to heat. In such cases you will observe that Point No. 28 of Adrenal when pressed would be paining. Common cold is often misunderstood and it is supressed by drugs (creating more heat in the body). There is a temporary relief, but as soon as the body becomes healthy, it tries to throw out excess water from the system and again diagnosed as a case of common cold. When such a phenomenon continues, it is declared as an allergy. The patient becomes a chronic case of sinusitis, tonsilitis, allergy and sometimes asthma. Later on, such patients get arthritis, rheumatism, etc.

In all the cases, it is surprising to observe that the lungs of the patient are clear in the beginning and only after continued chronic cold, are they sometimes affected and this leads to asthma.

A lady had asthma for 20 years. On examination, Point No. 28 of her, Adrenal was found damaged. As such, she was put on treatment for cold due to heat. In the beginnig the cold increased. She continued treatment and along with the same she took 2/3 glasses of lukewarm gold/silver/copper charged water and to her own surprise she got rid of this chronic problem in just 40 days.

**This method of diagnosis is a very unique feature of this therapy.** It helps you to locate a developing disease even before its outward symptoms appear. For example, if you have eaten or drunk anything which contained germs of jaundice, the liver gets damaged and within 48 hours or less, you can find that the point related to liver (Point No. 23) is paining. Now, jaundice normally is traced in blood after 4 days and in urine after five to seven days. **An early diagnosis**

**of any disease is always the most important factor for its cure.** You come to know what is wrong with you without any tests and can thus cure the disease at the earliest before it worsens in the body. **Such early detection is possible even for cancer and it is most necessary to control it. (For detailed stydy read author's book INSTANT DIAGNOSIS)**

( 3 ) **Cure :** As laymen, we are not much interested in knowing the name of the disease. We are more interested in getting rid of it once we diagnose it by the above method. The cure is very simple. After you have pressed your palms or soles for 10 minutes as a daily routine and located the points where it pains, you apply pressure intermittently like pumping for two minutes at a time only on the points where it pains. Repeat this treatment three times during 24 hours. **This treatment is to be continued only till you feel pain on that point. When the pain ceases, the disease is also removed with it and you are cured.** Then, this extra treatmen is to be stopped. As this therapy is based on bio-electricity, the relief is many times faster than even by injections. Therefore, sometimes the pain goes away within half to one minute.

**In case the symptoms of the disease initially aggravate during the treatment it is a clear sign that this treatment is working properly.** Nature wants to remove the disease from the body and so when you take this treatment, sometimes the symptoms initially aggravate. For example, when you have cold and headache, you will find pain on Point Nos. 1 to 7 and 34. When you take treatment by pressing them, the congested water is thrown out of the body, so the nose may start running or you may start sneezing. But once the root cause is removed, the cold will be cured very soon.

In the case of a chronic disease, you will start getting some relief improvement within 8 to 10 days and with continued treatment the illness will be completely cured.

**The motto of Acupressure is : If you feel pain, press it out.**

**Position :** Treatment can be taken in any position convenient to you i.e. while sitting, lying, standing or even travelling. Theretore, no special time is needed for taking this treatment. This treatment can be taken by the patient himself or can be given by others. For example, children or invalids can be given this treatment by parents or other family members *(See fig. 51)*.

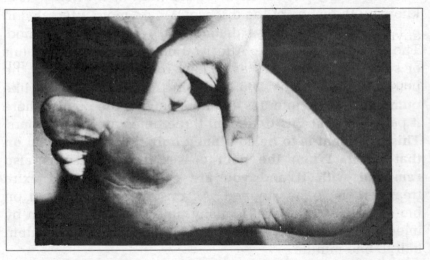

**Fig. 51 : Picture showing how pressure can be applied by others**

**Limitation :** Most of the diseases are cured with this natural treatment. However, if you do not find even 15 % improvement after taking the treatment for 12 to 15 days, it indicates that the damage/illness is severe and that you are in need of further assistance by way of change in diet, medical assistance or even hospitalisation.

**Time :** Though this treatment can be taken any time during the 24 hours of a day, it is advisable to avoid it for one hour after meals.

**Side Effects : An important positive feature of this treatment is that there are no side effects.** The treatment is harmless and can be safely given even to a one day old child. **As there are no side effects, you can take this treatment as a daily routine and make it a life style.**

You will discover the following by making this treatment a regular habit :

( 1.) All the organs will be recharged and all the endocrine glands will be controlled, thus leading to the proper functioning of the body and reducing the possibility of illness.

( 2 ) You will get a free daily medical check-up and anything wrong in your body will by found out immediately.

( 3 ) You can cure the disease at the earliest. Thus you become your Own Doctor.

( 4 ) You will be free not only from minor diseases like cold, headache, cough etc. but also from dreaded diseases like cancer, heart-attack, blood pressure, paralysis, diabetes, etc. **The net result will be that you will enjoy perfect Health.**

**Anaesthetic Effect :** If continued pressure on any point is applied for more than three minutes, it creates an anaesthetic effect on the organ connected with it. If the points

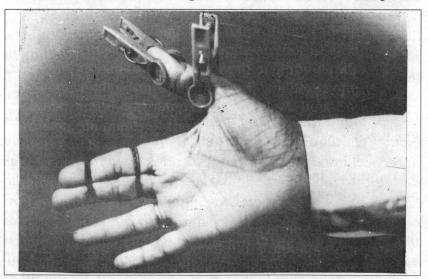

Fig. 52 : Picture showing how to use clothes-clips or
rubber bands to create an anaesthetic effect

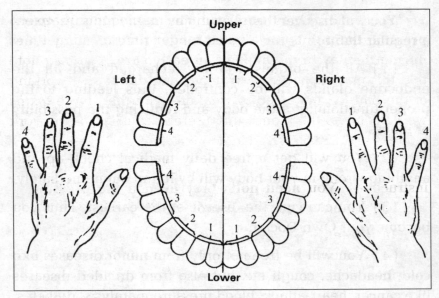

**Fig. 53 : Picture showing which finger is to be pressed
continuously for removing toothache in different teeth**

are on fingers, clothes-clips or rubber bands can be used as
shown in fig. 52. In case the tips of fingers or toes become
blue, this pressure should be removed. Such continued
pressure on corresponding points is very useful during severe
headache, stomach-ache, etc. For toothache, continuous
pressure is to be applied on the tips of the fingers relating to
that particular tooth *(See fig. 52 & 53).*

Dr 'M' reports : *I went to an exhibition. In one of the
stalls, I found the proprietor sitting in a corner, pressing his
mouth. On inquiry, I learnt that he had a severe toothache
in the last lower tooth of the right side. I told him that I was
a Medical Practitioner and asked him to press the tip of the
last finger continuously for five minutes. Afterwards, I went
away and came back after about an hour. I had to search for
the fellow who was very busy with his customers. He saw me
and came running to tell me that his toothache had gone
completely and he felt that God had sent me there with a
special purpose.*

**Precaution : It is observed that many people go on pressing the points for a much longer time or many times during the day in the hope of an early cure.** You may note that this may damage the switches and due to overworking of the battery, may lead to weakness. Further, more toxins would come to the kidney and thereby cause it to overwork which sometimes might damage it.

You must study the diagrams properly and follow the instructions. **You need not worry even if the pressure is applied around the point and not exactly on it.**

**Instruments :** A well known Acupressurist of U.S.A. with a practice of over 50 years, writes that **the best instruments are the thumbs and the fingers.** In the picture below, a few handy instruments like – hand massager, wooden clips, rubber bands, copper wire, aluminium combs and wooden roller with grooves, are shown. Costly instruments like fancy wooden rollers, sandals, mats, etc. are not considered to be necessary. These instruments only activate the organs in general, but Diagnosis or Cure is not possible with their help. Moreover, their excessive use may be harmful.

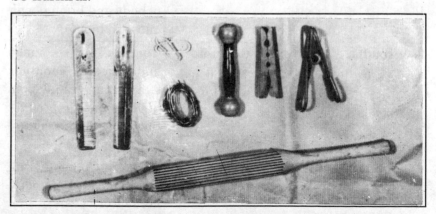

Fig. 54 : Picture showing handy devices like clothes-pin, rubber band, wooden stick, copper wire and grooved wooden rolling pin

# CHAPTER 4

# ENDOCRINE GLANDS – REGULATORS OF THE BODY

Nature has provided the body with proper regulators and protectors. These are the endocrine glands. The knowledge so far available in the west about these ductless endocrine glands in very limited. However, yogis in India were aware of their great importance, working and even before Ayurved – 6000 years and have described them as chakras.

| Name of Chakra | Equivalent Endocrine Gland | Its Working |
|---|---|---|
| 1. Sahastrar | Pineal *(Point No. 4)* | Regulates water balance; acts as a manager of all the glands; controls cerebro spinal fluid and sex desire. Stimulates growth of nerves. |
| 2. Ajna | Pituitary *(Point No. 3)* | Controls air and space. It is like king of all glands : controls growth of body and brain power and also memory. |
| 3. Vishudha | Thyroid/Parathyroid *(Point No. 8)* | Controls air – so lungs and heart; controls temperature regulation; governs energy production through the control of calcium. |
| 4. Anahat | Thymus *(Point No. 38)* | Acts as a Godmother till child reaches puberty i.e. 12 to 15 years of age. |

| Name of Chakra | Equivalent Endocrine Gland | Its Working |
|---|---|---|
| 5. Manipur | Adrenal and Pancreas *(Point No. 28 & Point No. 25)* | Controls fire and production of digestive juices. Regulates blood and sugar levels; controls stress-activeness and character building; controls sodium and water balance. |
| 6. Swadhis-than | Solar Plexus *(Point No. 29)* | Controls Apan Vayu "(अपान वायु)" and so regulates the movement of stools and urine; also controls all organs below the diaphragm. |
| 7. Mooladhar | Sex/gonads *(Point No. 11 to 15)* | Controls water and phosphorous content – Produces sex hormones. |

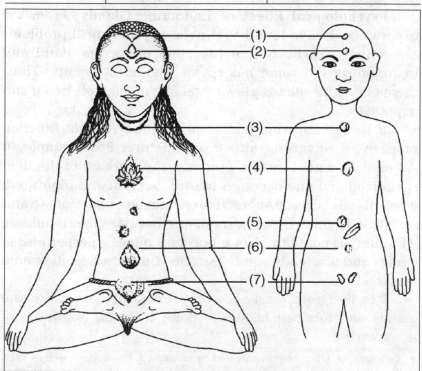

Fig. 55

These main endocrine glands produce internal secretions which on getting mixed with the blood, go to build up the body and maintain it in a healthy condition. The yogis have shown that these endocrine glands – (chakras) also mould the mind and character. In the second chapter, it is narrated that with certain yogic exercises, the latent electricity lying at the bottom can be moved upwards and the power of these endocrine glands can be increased manifold.

The main function of these glands is to maintain the metabolism – (control of the five basic elements (shown in chapter II)) of the body; regulate the functions of all the organs and the brain; also to adjust the body against changing environment and thus protect the body against any illness. These glands play a very important role not only in the development of our body and mind, but also in the development of our looks and even character.

**Psychological Effect of Endocrine Glands :** From my experience, I have found that even psychological problems are connected with one or the other endocrine gland and treatment of the same has given wonderful results. Thus, these endocrine glands play a vital role in our well-being and happiness.*

If these endocrine glands of our body do not function properly, it adversely affects our nature. For example, if Adrenal does not function properly, the working of the liver is affected and one becomes fearful, peevish and illnatured; if Sex glands become overactive one becomes passionate and selfish; if Thymus is not normal, one becomes meanminded; if Pituitary is not normal, one becomes pitiless, perpetrator of crimes and this leads one to become a thief, a dacoit, even a murderer.

It is, therefore, most necessary to control these endocrine glands and this can be easily done with the treatment of Acupressure.

---

* Very recently it has been discovered by urologist J. Edwin Blackwell in 1979, that all the systems of our body can be kept functioning properly by activiting the exocrine and endocrine glands.

**Endocrine Glands :** There are seven endocrine glands in the body. They are interrelated and dependent on one another and assist one another. **So while treating one gland, it is necessary to treat other glands.** In case of any problem for about eight to ten days, you will find that there is a pain on *(Point No. 8)* of Thyroid/Parathyroid. **They are the barometers of the body.** In case of chronic problems, you will observe that points of more than one endocrine gland would be paining.

**Thymus Gland (Point No. 38) :** This is a very important gland and can be considered as a God-Mother for the child. It protects the growing young child against any disease. If treatment is given for two minutes twice a day on the point of this gland in the soles till the child is of one year and then also in the two palms till the age of 12/15 years along with treatment on points of all other endocrine glands and organs, the child will grow and develop properly in body and mind.

Once the body is fully developed, this gland shrinks and stops its activities. However, if for some reason, it becomes active, it produces dullness and general fatigue leading to total inactiveness. (Known as Myasthenia). The point of this gland is situated under Point No. 30 and as such, deeper pressure is to be applied on Point No. 30 to reach the Point No. 38 of Thymus gland.

**Thyroid/Parathyroid Glands (Point No. 8) :** These glands play an important role in the development of the child's body. As they digest calcium and eliminate poison, toxins, they assist in controlling of the heat of the body and thus maintain the child's health. If these glands do not function properly, it leads to weakness, diseases even twisting of muscles, leading to rickets and convulsions and so the development of a child is retarded. The child becomes fat and dull. Similarly, the overworking of this gland leads to overgrowth, bulging eyes, goitre, protruding Adam's apple and tendency to become a bully. Even after puberty, if this gland does not function properly, it leads to problem of calcification(stone). This gland controls the element of air and so the lungs and the heart.

It also helps build human qualities like affection, love, capacity for high thinking and concentration leading to self control and balanced temperament, purity of heart and unselfishness. When it is deranged, a person becomes mentally unsteady, too talkative and ungrateful. When this gland is damaged along with sex glands; women, during pregnancy and or after child birth or removal of ovaries, tend to become plumpy and put on weight around the abdomen and waist.

*Mr. 'V' reports about two patients discharged from a reputable hospital in Mumbai as being incurable. They were found to be suffering from toxic Thyroid and were given Acupressure treatment. On the 4th day, both the patients showed signs of improvement and within 40 days, they were completely cured.*

As these glands are the barometers of the body, there is a pain on their Point No. 8 when there is a complaint of over 8/10 days. They play a vital role in our health and happiness and as such their points occupy a big place in our palm/sole. When these glands are not functioning adequately, there is a deficiency of calcium; so it is also necessary to make up deficiency of the body by taking calcium – (cal. phos + cal flour-biochemic medicines.)

**Ovary-Testes-Sex-Gonad Glands (Points No. 11–15) :** These glands maintain the unbroken chain of procreation. They also regulate water element and also nerves, cells, flesh, bones, bonemarrow and semen. They also regulate digestion of phosphorous in the body and thus regulate heat of the body.

**Effects of Malfunctioning of Sex Glands :** Malfunctioning of these glands is noticeable only when children start getting mature at the age of 12 to 14. Girls have problems of menstruation(late or painful or too little) leading to pimples and excess heat in the body; or sometimes too much bleeding leading to anaemia. This leads to under development in the growth of the body.

As for boys, they turn to self-abuse, masturbation, start getting erotic dreams, become shy, often disturbing the growth of body and beard. Moreover, this creates psychological problems, which if not tackled immediately, many a time, become the root cause of unhappiness in couples in their early married life.

A regular and proper functioning of these glands helps in maintaining the heat of the body and plays an important role in contributing to the attractiveness of a boy or a girl. Moreover, their nature becomes amiable. They become charming with good manners and agreeable words and they enjoy a fine health. Its disorder makes one selfish, envious – censorious – lustful and of angry disposition.

After delivery and operation for sterilisation if these glands function less, fat starts accumulating in the body. So, to maintain proper figure of the body, women are advised to take treatment on their Points No. 14 and 15 during and after pregnancy. Further, these glands secrete sex hormones. Insufficient working creates rigidity and problems during menopause. Sometimes, the root cause for not bearing a child can be traced to the damaged condition of these sex glands of the couple.

*'A doctor couple had no issue even after 14 years of their marriage. Both of them started treatment on the points of these glands and within 15 months, they became proud parents of a baby girl.'*

**Pancreas Glands (Point No. 25) :** These glands regulate digestion of sugar – glucose in the body by creating insulin. In modern times due to excessive use of sugar, (not the natural sugar in cereals-fruits-milk-honey-which is easily digestable) it has become more necessary to look after the proper functioning of this gland.

Further, as per the latest research, it has been observed that overfunctioning of this gland leads to low B.P., Migraine and at times creates more desire for sweet food leading to diabetes and sweet drinks leading sometimes even to alcoholism.

*Mrs. G, wife of an Income tax officer, had severe Migraine for several years. She started taking Acupressure treatment and within 15 days she was completely cured.*

*Mr. P, an Acupressurist, observed that Pancreas gland was overworking in sixty workers who had been alcoholics. He showed them how to take treatment. More than 70% of the workers stopped taking alcohol.*

**Adrenal Glands (Point No. 28) :** This gland controls and regulates the fire element of the body and so controls spleen, liver and gall bladder and assists in the creation of biles and digestive juices. Qualities like keenness of perception, untiring activity, the drive to action, inner energy and courage are due to proper functioning of this gland. It also intensifies the flow of blood, helps proper oxygenation and develops organising power, leads to leadership. It plays an important part in character building of a child.

In case of disorder of this gland, persons abuse their natural vigour to satisfy their lust or antisocial activities. They suffer from a sense of vain glory and are conceited, become extremely restless, impatient and short tempered. They cannot control diet and suffer from stomach problems and blood pressure. Such persons become fearful, timid and lose vigour to face problems of life.

*A prince had lost interest in life from the age of 16. He stopped studies in the final year at the University and had no interest even in sex. So he did not marry. At the age of 31, after he unsuccessfully tried the treatment under various therapies, he consulted an Acupressurist. On examination it was found that his Thyroid and Adrenal glands had been damaged. The Acupressurist told that the cause of all his troubles was some type of deep fear, a severe shock which had damaged his Adrenal gland. The father of the prince admitted that the prince had, at the age of 16, joined him in hunting in a jungle and had fallen down from the horse and was miraculously saved from a tiger, and since then had suffered from hallucinations and lost interest in life. He was given Acupressure treatment and gold / silver / copper charged water to drink. Within 30 days he became normal and started taking interest in his hobby of painting and also in household chores.*

**Pituitary Gland (Point No. 3) :** This gland controls air and space in the body. This gland is like a king of all glands and sends orders to all other glands. It controls will-power, sight, hearing, memory and sanse of discrimination. It also rectifies the faults of other glands.

When it is predominant, it helps people to become great geniuses, eminent literary men, poets, scientists, philosophers and lovers of mankind.

As this gland controls the growth of the body, its overworking leads to make people physically big in size, while its insufficient functioning may result in making them dwarfs.

This gland also governs the growth of the mind-brain. This gland may be damaged due to fear or injury or sometimes, due to tension during pregnancy. This also leads to the malfunctioning of other glands. And that results in giving birth to mentally retarded children. So, if this problem of mentally retarded children is to be solved, the pregnant women during their pregnancy should take treatment on all endocrine glands and avoid damage to foetus. Further, it is observed that in those children where this gland is not working sufficiently, they tend to become mean, heartless, mischievous, tend to become bullies, liars and disobedient. They are even ready to steal. With proper treatment of this gland, in most cases the parents and teachers will get amazing results. As this gland and the Pineal gland are situated in the head, it is harmful to hit the children on the head.

*A 16 year old girl of a well-to-do family was reported to be stealing petty things of her classmates and no amount of persuasion, scolding or even corporal punishment had any effect on her. An Acupressurist found that the point of her*

*Pituitary gland was tender and on further examination her sex glands were also found to be damaged. On enquiry, she admitted that she had scanty as well as painful menses which was the root cause of her habit of stealing. She started taking, Acupressure treatment and within 15 days, she stopped stealing and within 45 days, her menses became normal.*

If the growth of the body and brain is not normal, give treatment on Point No. 3 in the middle of thumbs and big toes, to give necessary stimulation.

This gland could be damaged during pregnancy and child birth, which can lead to malfunctioning of other glands especially sex glands which in turn can lead to obesity after childbirth. All these prove the necessity of maintaining this gland in proper working condition.

**Pineal Gland (Point No. 4) :** It acts as an organiser and controller of all glands. It controls the development of the glands and regulates them. Malfunctioning of this gland leads to high B. P., awakening of premature sex glands and even sex delinquency. Moreover, it controls the Potassium/Sodium balance in the body and so its malfunctioning leads to excessive retention of fluids in the body which is mistaken for a serious kidney problem. It controls the proper flow of Cerebro Spinal Fluid and thus keeps all the glands and body vitalised, strong and healthy.

It is also known as a primitive third eye. The predominance of this gland generates a sense of sublimity helping men grow into saints, endowed with divine qualities. These people have great wisdom and tenderness of heart, but also strong will power and so are not affected by physical sufferings or sorrow.

**Lymph Glands (Point No. 16) :** Although they are not endocrine glands, because of their importance, they have been included here. The points of these glands are under Point No. 16 in the middle of the wrists. They control the immune defence system of our body, prevent the formation of pus on any cut or boil on the body and quickly heal the wounds.

These glands help clear the toxins from the body, clear the dead cells from the system. But when such toxins and dead cells are in excess in the body, these glands have to overwork and so, they become weak and tender. At such time, when you press on the point of these glands, it pains. If such pain continues, it means that these glands are not able to stop the malignant growth forming from toxins and dead cells. As such, the first symptom to detect cancer even at a very early stage is to find out about any pain on this gland. Moreover, during recent observation, it has also been found that if there is a pain on these glands and also on points of Pancreas, it indicates diabetes, increase of glucose in the blood. Thus, you will observe that to prevent cancer and sugar in blood, it is most necessary to keep these glands in an active condition.

**Increasing the Will-Power :** Our mind has a great effect on these glands. For example, continuous fear damages the Pituitary gland and makes one timid. Similarly, tension and worry disturb the Pineal gland and so leads to high B.P. and as Pineal gland controls other glands it also disturbs other glands and digestive system. In modern times, stress-tension or worry-fear have increased and they often disturb these endocrine glands. If these endocrine glands are not treated immediately, it might lead to malfunctioning of other glands of the body. As these glands are interrelated, whenever one gland is disturbed, the other glands also get disturbed. So, when you press on the points of these endocrine glands you will feel pain on points of more than one gland especially in case of chronic diseases. Therefore, it is very important to give treatment on all the endocrine glands and keep them under proper control.

These glands also control the mind (the will-power). So in order to get rid of bad habits like smoking, drinking, drug addiction or even overeating, it is extremely necessary to give treatment on all the endocrine glands for at least, fifteen days. Because, these people lack the necessary will-power to give up bad habits, they often break their vows to stop such bad habits and so they are considered unreliable. However, a treatment of fifteen days will give them necessary will-power to stop these bad habits after that. And they will be free from the withdrawal symptoms of stopping these bad habits.

*A Government officer had the habit of drinking alcohol every evening. He started Acupressure treatment and drank hot water in the evening instead. Surprisingly, he succeeded in getting rid of his habit of drinking.*

*A young man was addicted to drugs in spite of many persuasions by his mother and brother. He continued breaking vows and taking drugs. He was advised Acupressure treatment and so after one month he got himself free not only from drugs but also from smoking and even masturbation.*

**It has been observed that if children are taught to take this treatment from an early age of 8–10; not only will their physical growth be normal but they will have no problems at the time of puberty and inclination towards delinquency and they will become attractive and will develop a well balanced outlook on life and will be able to live happily as good citizens.**

If the police–crime department tries this treatment on the juveniles and criminals, it will be possible to reduce the crime rate.

**Psychological Problems : Many problems, considered to be psychological are a result of improper functioning of the endocrine glands.** So, with proper treatment on the glands such problems can be easily solved.

**Case study :** *A girl with a bright record in school, had at the age of 17, a typical problem. About 45 days before the examination, her hands started shivering five minutes after she started reading and the book would fall down. So she was not able to prepare for examination and day by day she became more and more nervous. An Acupressurist was consulted. Her Adrenal gland was tender-damaged. On* *further examination her sex glands were also found to have been disturbed. On being asked whether she had profuse bleeding before this complaint started, she agreed. She started taking Acupressure treatment and in due course passed the examination creditably.*

*A young Professor came to our centre one day (Wednesday) morning and informed me that he was so much depressed that he desired to commit suicide. Jokingly, I agreed that he should commit suicide on next Wednesday evening at 3.00 p.m. But meanwhile, he should take the treatment on all endocrine glands and drink charged water during the week and report to me on next Wednesday morning. Then he came with a smiling face only to inform that he wanted to live long and enjoy life. His desire to commit suicide had disappeared. Similarly, thousands of cases can be quoted.*

It has been admitted by Allopathic practitioners that by taking unnatural hormones like estrogen to counter the effects of menopause, the possibility of developing cancer in the body greatly increases. The best way to control hormonal balance, is to take treatment on Point No. 11 to 15 atleast twice a day. It will ensure that this natural phenomenon of menopause passes away without any side effects. Moreover, when Sex glands are disturbed, Thyroid and Parathyroid glands are also disturbed, leading either to decalcification or leading to fracture or forming of stones. As such, treatment on Point No. 8 and other endocrine glands is necessary.

It has been observed that in case of the cancer, as the disease progresses, these endocrine glands become more and more tender, and because of overworking, they become tired and eventually stop secreting the most vital hormones in the body and damage the very metabolism of the body and at this stage this disease is considered malignant, and if proper treatment is not taken, it develops rapidly and becomes deadly. **Hence, the great necessity of controlling all the endocrine glands must be properly realised.** If all the endocrine glands are controlled properly and thereby all the organs, the possibility of cancer becomes remote.

**In case of severe damage due to overworking / underworking of any of the endocrine glands, i.e., hypothyroid; same treatment as mentioned for cancer on pages 238 to 241 is to be taken.**

It is only the Acupressure therapy which shows the proper way to control these vital glands in the easiest way. As all the endocrine glands are inter-related, in order to correct the defects of one gland, it is necessary to give treatment on all the endocrine glands. These glands are situated deep inside the body and so a little more pressure preferably with the thumb in a vertical position or unsharpened pencil or harder massage on the same will be necessary.

### Functions and Effects of the Malfunctioning of Endocrine Glands

| Name of the Gland | Effect of Malfunctioning |
| --- | --- |
| **1. Thymus Gland (Point No. 38)** Protects the child up to the age of 15. | Child gets sick. In case this gland becomes active later on, it brings dullness. |
| **2. Pineal Gland (Point No. 4)** Controls sex system and water of body and is a primitive eye. | Premature sex development, increase in water content, high B. P. |
| **3. Pituitary Gland (Point No. 3)** It is the king of glands and controls the other glands. Governs the brain and the development of the body. | Body becomes dwarfish or bulging. Produces mental retardation. Child becomes a bully, or a liar and disobedient. |

| Name of the Gland | Effect of Malfunctioning |
|---|---|
| **4. Thyroid & Para-thyroid Glands (Point No. 8)** Para-thyroid gland controls digestion of calcium in the body. Also controls the development of the body. | Underworking leads to rickets, convulsion, teeth problems, twisting of muscles, fatness and dullness. Overworking leads to over-growth, bulging of the eyes. Adam's apple, stone in the kidney, etc. |
| **5. Adrenal Gland (Point No. 28)** Controls production of biles and controls the liver and the flow of blood, B.P. and also moulds character. | Underworking leads to dullness, timidness, less energy, less oxygenation. Overworking leads to high B.P. migrane headache. Less biles lead to acidity and vomitting and severe headache. |
| **6. Pancreas (Point No. 25)** Controls digestion of sugar in the body, and digestive juices. | Underworking leads to diabetes and overworking leads to low B.P., dizziness and even to alcoholism through Hypoglycemia i.e. shortage of sugar. |
| **7. Ovaries, Testes & Sex Glands (Point No. 14 & 15)** Controls digestion of phosphorus and heat of the body, attractiveness and productive side of life. | Reproductive organs are damaged, problems of less or more menses, self-abuse, loss of heat leading to development of fat, un-attractiveness of the body, less/more sex desire. |
| **8. Lymph Gland (Point No. 16)** Stops formation of pus and prevents germs. | Disease called Lymphocytosis. Leads to increase in blood-sugar. |

# CHAPTER 5

# ROOT CAUSES AND ERADICATION OF DISEASES

The treatment under Acupressure therapy is based on the assumption that you are taking a balanced diet i.e. a diet containing seasonal fruits, green vegetables, proteins, carbohydrates, fats, minerals and vitamins in proper proportions. Any disease caused by the deficiency in such most required food for the body CANNOT BE CURED WITHOUT SUPPLEMENTING THE DIET. For Indians, normal food of chapati or roti, vegetables, cereals, occasional rice, milk or curd or buttermilk and seasonal fruits will form quite a balanced diet. In the same way, the diet of Europeans and Americans is also balanced except that they should reduce the use of fine flour, coffee (which causes constipation) and sugar.

As explained in the third chapter, all the organs of the body can be activated or recharged by Acupressure treatment. Almost all the parts of the body except lungs and stomach are autonomous and will function well so long as they get enough oxygen and proper blood supply. That is why lungs (respiratory system) and stomach (the digestive system) play the most important role in the functioning of the body. It is quite likely that germs of a disease enter our body through them.

**Respiratory System :**

**Lungs :** From childhood, proper care of breathing and expansion of lungs should be taken. Outdoor games, running and laughing and even crying by children, give enough scope for the expansion of their lungs. However, pranayam should be taught from childhood, from the age of 5/6 years for proper breathing for proper oxygenation and purification of blood.

**Pranayam – The Easy way :** While sitting or lying straight,

| | |
|---|---|
| Inhale air counting | 1-2-3-4... |
| then keep the air in the lungs counting | 1-2-3-4.... |
| and then exhale counting | 1-2-3-4. |
| Then pause. Do not inhale counting. | 1-2-3-4. |

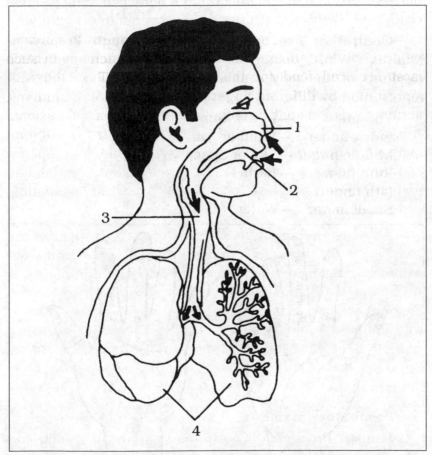

Fig. 56 : 1. Nose. 2. mouth. 3. windpipe. 4. lungs (Point No. 30)

Please repeat this atleast 10 to 15 times. Do such Pranayam 4 to 10 times a day and with practice go on increasing the counting to about 10. During the pause only, the lungs get rest and are revitalised. This type of controlled breathing, called Pranayam, was tried on T.B. patients in a hospital in Chicago and the results were astounding.

**Pranayam :** Once you reach counting 10 you may develop Pranayam as under :

| | |
|---|---|
| Inhale counting | (up to) 10 |
| Retain counting | (up to) 20 |
| Exhale counting | (up to) 10 |
| Refrain from in haling, counting | (up to) 10 |
| i.e. in the ratio of | 1:2:1:1 |

**Control of five basic elements through Pranayam-Mudras :** While doing this Pranayam, even five basic elements of the body can be controlled because they are represented by different fingers as under :

| | |
|---|---|
| Thumb | —Fire or Sun |
| Index finger | —Wind or Air |
| Middle finger | —Sky or Space |
| Ring finger | —Earth |
| (4th finger) | |
| Small finger | —Water |

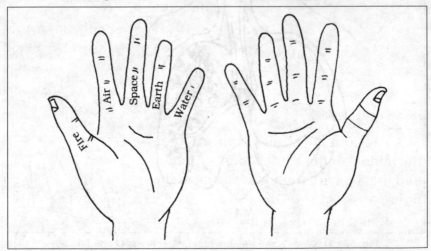

Fig. 57 : Five fingers represent five elements

Now, through different combinations of these fingers–mudras, we can not only control these elements but also cure many diseases. This can be done in any position but sitting in a lotus position or sukhasan is advisable for better results. They can be started in 10 minutes and performed for at least

30 to 45 minutes. **Some of such mudras are shown below and are to be performed with both hands simultaneously.**

**( 1 ) Meditation Mudra :** Simply touch the thumb with index finger– pressing is not neccessary.

**Benefits :** This helps in increasing brain power, mental concentration, memory, etc. and cures problems of sleeplessness, tension, lack of concentration.

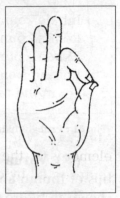

Fig. 58 :
Meditation Mudra

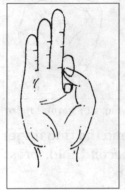

Fig. 59 : Vayu Mudra

**( 2 ) Vayu Mudra (Air) :** Keep the index finger on the base of the thumb at the mount of Venus and press with the thumb as shown in the figure.

**Benefits :** It cures rheumatism, artharitis, gout, Parkinson's disease and blood circulation problems. For better results, also do Pran Mudra.

**( 3 ) Shunya Mudra (Space) :** Keep the middle finger at the mount of Venus and press it with thumb as shown in the figure.

**Benefits :** It helps in curing earache, deafness, vertigo, etc. It is necessary to do this Mudra for 40 to 60 minutes to get the best results.

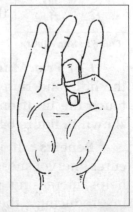

Fig. 60 : Shunya Mudra

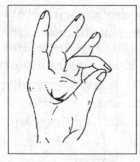

Fig. 61 : Prithvi Mudra

**(4) Prithvi Mudra (Earth) :** Put the ring finger together with the thumb as shown in figure 61.

**Benefits :** It cures weakness of the body and the mind. It increases life force, (chetana) and gives new vigour to an ailing person. It also gives peace of mind.

**(5) Varun Mudra (Water) :** Put the tips of thumb and little finger together as shown in figure 62.

**Benefits :** It cures impurities of blood, skin problems and makes the skin smooth. Useful in gastro-enteritis and any other disease causing dehydration.

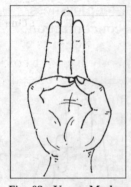

Fig. 62 : Varun Mudra

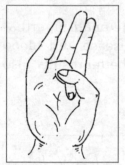

Fig. 63 : Sun Mudra

**(6) Sun Mudra :** Bend the ring finger and on its outer side on second fold, press with thumb as per figure 63.

**Benefits :** It creates heat in the body, helps digestion and helps in reducing fat in the body.

**(7) Pran Mudra (Life Energy) :** Bend the little and ring fingers so that their tips touch the tip (front edge) of the thumb as shown in figure 64.

**Benefits :** It increases life force and cures nervousness, and fatigue. It also helps increasing power of the eyes and in reducing the number of glasses (spectacles).

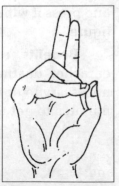

Fig. 64 : Pran Mudra

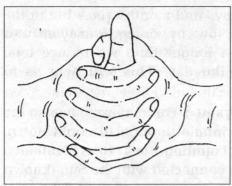

**Fig. 65 : Ling Mudra**

**( 8 ) Ling      (Shiv) Mudra :** Join both the palms and interlock the fingers. Keep the thumb of the left hand vertically straight and encircle it with the index finger and the thumb of right hand as shown in figure 65.

**Benefits :** It increases the power of resistance of the body against cold and bronchial infections and also against changes in weather, fever due to cold. It gives power to the lungs, creates heat in the body and burns up accumulated phlegm and even fat. While practicing this mudra one must drink plenty of green and fruit juices and water, at least 8 glasses a day.

Now, while performing these mudras if Pranayam is done, you will get better results.

**Retention of Air :** While doing Pranayam, after inhaling air press the upper part of the Thumb no. 1 with the index finger. You will be able to retain air easily in the lungs for a longer time than without such locking *(See figure 66)*.

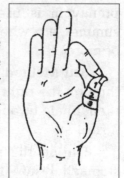

Fig. 66

Now if, the middle of the thumb No. 2 is pressed, the retention increases. See fig. 66. Now if the base of the thumb (No. 3) is pressed, the retention is maximum.

**How to Increase Longevity :** If there is more retention of air in lungs, it is fully utilised, gives better power to blood and body. This will also mean that less breaths are taken. According to Indian philosophy, our life span is fixed and is measured not in minutes, days and months/years but in the total number of breaths. Now by doing Pranayam and retaining air in lungs for a longer time we reduce total number of breaths during the day. **This will help us to increase our longevity.**

**1st Method (Sun Pranayam) :** For increasing heat in the body, close the left nostril, inhale through the right nostril and exhale through it whilst counting 1 to 4/10 as mentioned above. As the right nostril is connected with the Sun (known as Pingala Nadi in Yoga) inhaling and exhaling through it will produce heat in the body. Therefore, such pranayam is very useful in winter and monsoon and for diseases like cold, asthma, polio, paralysis, bronchitis, arthritis, T.B., etc. wherein heat is required. Do this ten times or more.

**2nd Method (Moon Pranayam) :** For increasing coolness in the body, close the right nostril, inhale and exhale through the left nostril whilst counting as above. The left nostril is connected with the moon (known as Ida in Yoga). So, it produces coolness in the body. Therefore, such pranayam is useful in diseases like fever, sunstroke in summer, etc. wherein coolness is necessary. Do this ten times or more.

**3rd Method (For balancing of heat and cold) :** Inhale through the right nostril and exhale from the left nostril and then inhale through the left nostril and exhale from the right nostril.

During the period the breath is held inside, pull the stomach inside for more effective results as well as for reducing the tummy.

Please see to it that while inhaling, your chest should expand by 5 to 7 cm. Better results can be obtained by breathing as above. Pranayam can be done in a comfortable posture, by sitting upright on the ground or a chair/sofa or can be done in a standing position or even while walking.

Breathing from the desired nostril–right or left–can be effected by closing the other nostril. Otherwise, if you lie down on the left side of the body, the breath will flow from the right nostril. In India people are advised to lie down for 10 to 15 minutes on the left side after lunch or dinner so that the breath is linked with the sun, producing heat in the body and helping digestion. Similarly, if you lie down on the right side, the breath will flow from the left nostril which is useful during too much heat or fever.

**4th Method (Kapalbhati) :** Sit upright in a quiet place. Inhale and exhale very fast through the nostrils. Start with 10 times and go up to 50 times in a minute. Do this pranayam for 2 minutes/twice a day.

**5th Method (Bhastrika) :** Open the mouth, inhale slowly through it and then immediately blow out hard through nostrils. Do it for 10 to 15 times. Do this pranayam every time after you do Kapalbhati. That will clear up congestion in the head.

Regular practice of pranayam and breathing exercises will ensure proper oxygenation of all parts of the body and cure many diseases. Proper oxygenation helps in purifying the blood and removal of toxins and carbon dioxide from the body. This, in turn, will reduce the unnecessary burden on kidney, reducing the possibility of skin diseases and failure of kidney. Moreover, pure blood enables proper functioning of all the organs and thereby increases vigour and vitality.

These breathing exercises are beneficial to all and should be practised daily. However, these exercises are a must for the treatment of cold, cough, asthma, T.B. and mental disorders like polio, meningitis, nervous breakdown, muscular distrophy, etc.

**Time :** Pranayam should be done on an empty stomach or two hours after meals. Mudras can be done any time.

**Digestive System :** For good health, formation of pure blood is most important. Pure blood is formed from the food and drink we take and digest. Therefore, it is necessary to give proper attention to our digestive system.

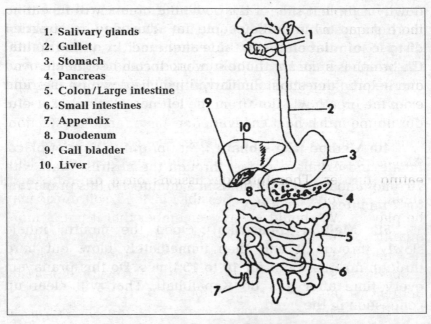

1. Salivary glands
2. Gullet
3. Stomach
4. Pancreas
5. Colon/Large intestine
6. Small intestines
7. Appendix
8. Duodenum
9. Gall bladder
10. Liver

Fig. 67 : Digestive system

All the cells of our body get changed within a cycle of seven years. So, by changing our diet, we can change the whole system – even Prakruti of our body. Thus a weakling or a patient suffering from a chronic disease can become strong and healthy with necessary change in diet and exercise.

*"The case of Mr. Bernar Macfaden of U.S.A. is very illustrative. He got T.B. at an early age of seventeen. The doctors lost all hope of curing him. He changed his diet completely. He began taking only fruits and vegetables. He started nature cure treatment including fasting, sunbath exercises, etc. What he achieved was almost a miracle."*

Please note that care of our digestive system should start from the mouth. Nature has given us teeth to chew. Therefore, we should form the habit of chewing all food including liquid food and soft food like sweets, ice-creams, etc. at least 12 to 15 times. This is necessary to add saliva to the food, for it is only in saliva that the sugar is digested. That is why people eating hastily without chewing and eating more sugar invite diabetes and fat. **The modern dreaded disease of diabetes can be conquered in your mouth.** Chewing less means double work for the stomach. And over-exertion of the stomach will invite many diseases and even fat.

Proper chewing gives better taste and satisfaction. Moreover, it enables you to listen to Nature's signal that your stomach has become full. This in turn enables you to stop eating further. Therefore, discussions on a dinning table should be avoided as far as possible. Instead, soft music may be played. We should always remember that it is not more quantity or heavy food but the food that is digested that gives us energy. If everybody forms the habit of chewing food properly, less food will be necessary which will incidentally help in solving the problem of food scarcity.

**Diet :** The aim of eating and drinking should be to produce enough blood, produce sufficient heat and energy in the body and satisfy the taste.

There are six types of tastes : (1) sweet, (2) salty, (3) sour, (4) hot (chilly), (5) astringent and (6) bitter.

It has been observed that we avoid more and more the last two types of taste with the result that it upsets the digestive system and balance in our blood, thereby leading to a number of diseases, including cancer. These tastes nullify the effect of sweets and purify the blood. These two tastes increase the digestive power (the fire) and are like a starter in a car and therefore should be included in our diet. It may be observed that Mahatma Gandhi insisted on paste of neem leaves (चटणी) in the daily diet. An English medical practitioner has observed that those Indian people who use neem leaves in their diet are healthier and are more immune to disease, including blood cancer than those who don't use them.

We take great care about the quality and quantity of coal or wood we put in the cooking furnace or fireplace. We also give it enough air to burn properly. This enables the fire to give maximum heat and reduce smoke and ashes to the minimum. We should not forget that there is a similar fireplace in our stomach. We must think of the after-effects of the food and drink we take. The difference in the proportion of three basic elements of water, fire and wood in our body depends upon the food we eat. As laymen, we should see that the fire in the stomach is well maintained so that the normal food is digested. After the age of 35, we should be able to know what type of food does not suit us. We should, therefore, avoid such unsuitable foods. We must know that a particular food which may be good for certain people may not be suitable to others e.g. curd/yoghurt, buttermilk suitable to people having more elements of fire, would not be suitable to people having more elements of water in them. Again, curd/yoghurt and buttermilk are advisable in the hot season, but not in the monsoon season.

**Easy way to find out what food/drink is suitable to oneself :** First stand straight, keep your left hand fist closed on the heart, outstretch your right hand parallel to the ground. Ask someone to pull down the right hand.

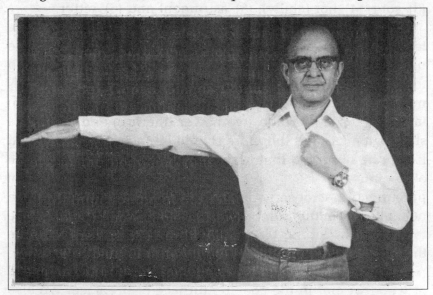

Fig. 68 : Picture showing how to find out what food/drink is suitable

Resist as much as possible. Now, keep the eatable in your left hand palm and keep it on your heart and outstretch your right hand parallel to the ground. Ask someone to pull down your right hand. Now if this eatable is beneficial to your body resistance power will increase. If it is harmful, resistance power will be greatly reduced and right hand will come down easily. In case of a drink you can keep it in a metal utensil preferably copper and do as shown above.

This method is based on the electricity of our body. Proper food/drink enhances the polarisation of electric flow and so increases the power of resistance. Improper food/drink depolarises the flow and so the resistance is reduced.

This way, you can find out easily what to eat and drink and what to avoid. Because of difference in the type of Prakruti, it is very possible that something suitable to someone may not be useful to another person. e.g. curd/yoghurt mixed with sugar will be found more suitable to persons having more fire (पित्त प्रकृति) but not to those persons having more of water+earth (कफ प्रकृति) and less of fire element. So everybody can try this method and find out what foods are useful and what foods are harmful to them. **This way one can find out which one drug, out of many similar drugs, would be more suitable to one.**

It will be observed by this method, that just to satisfy the taste, we eat so much useless things which do not generate energy, but in order to digest such useless foods our energy has to be used and still more energy has to be used to throw out such useless dead food which many a time produces gases, constipation, etc.

If we make a habit of eating and drinking only such things as are useful to our body and chew them properly the total requirement of food will be reduced considerably, digestion will improve and in the same way discharge of stool will be easy.

Thus, maximum energy will be obtained by the body from a minimum intake of food. If this principle is accepted by mankind on a larger scale, the total requirement of food will be less and there will be minimum health problems and famines.

**How to get maximum energy from the food :** Recent experiments by nutrition experts in the U.S.A. have confirmed the finding of the Indian philosophy that the best time to eat food is one hour after we get up in the morning till sunset when internal temperature increases and the food is digested more easily and so more energy is obtained. They have maintained that eating late and taking heavy foods after sunset, tend to slow down digestion and produces more fat and problems of the stomach.

In Ayurved, the Indian medical system, a detailed description of the after-effects of all the different types of cereals, vegetables, spices, fruits, milk, curd, buttermilk, herbs, minerals, etc. is given. This shows a deep study and research over hundreds of years. Ayurved describes minutely what food to eat, how to eat and when to eat and also shows the effective use of kitchen spices in curing certain diseases. It would be worth the effort to study the same and implement it. Out of so many important ingredients of the kitchen spices, one is turmeric (हलदी) powder. It is very useful as described below :

( 1 ) On any cuts, bleeding or burns, turmeric powder should be applied immediately. It is antiseptic and will stop bleeding and heal the cut / burn effectively.

( 2 ) Whenever there is pain in bones or swelling due to a fall, this powder is to be boiled in water and a thick paste has to be applied for 3 to 4 days on that swelling or the part that pains and cover it with a bandage; and without any other medication, the pain and the swelling will subside.

( 3 ) In case of Tonsillitis, apply a paste of this powder and glycerine tanic acid, massage on tonsils with the tip of the finger, and then gargle with lukewarm salt water. Do this for two to three days.

In the case of small children, if they do not allow such a massage, globules of the size of green peas may be made with this powder and jaggery and 8 to 12 pills a day be given to children.

( 4 ) Turmeric is blood purifier and so can be taken with milk. It should be given this way to the mother after delivery. This helps faster contraction of the ovaries and inner parts.

( 5 ) A paste of turmeric powder and sandalwood powder mixed with a little edible oil can be applied on your face as a face mask. Keep it for 15/20 minutes. Then wash your face with tap water. Within 15/20 days your face will look bright and radiant.

( 6 ) In diabetes, regular intake of turmeric powder and *Amla* powder has been found very effective.

Like turmeric, other spices are also useful in many ways. So we should learn about their usefulness and make use of them accordingly.

**To maintain a good digestive system we should see that —**

( 1 ) the food is well cooked and eaten warm / hot.

( 2 ) the use of whole wheat and rice is adequate. Please try to reduce or avoid use of fine flour and polished rice.

( 3 ) use of fried things is reduced.

( 4 ) enough buttermilk and curd are included in the diet.

( 5 ) enough vegetables, raw and cooked and seasonal fruits are taken.

( 6 ) the food is properly chewed.

( 7 ) a time gap of 5 to 7 hours is kept between two meals.

( 8 ) the habit of drinking liquids except water or buttermilk or eating between the meals is stringently controlled.

( 9 ) the stomach is given rest of at least one or two meals a week as it is a machine. At that time, only fruits or fruit juices or boiled water may be taken.

**Traffic Signal :** To satisfy our palate is one of the greatest enjoyments of life. Eat anything you like once in a while. But respect nature's signal which is given in the form of belching. Nature gives a first signal to say that the stomach is full. You should stop eating further at that point. It is an orange/amber signal like the one at the traffic lights. If that cannot be done, **You must stop at the second signal which is like a red light.** If you continue eating even after the second signal, please be warned that you are inviting trouble. Necessary changes in the food/diet, should be made according to the changes in the seasons.

Please observe the motto that the fire in the stomach should be well preserved and should remain capable of digesting the food you eat.

A liberal use of ginger, pepper, eatables of bitter taste, sunbath, regular exercise, etc. helps this fire, while cold water, cold drinks, icecream, etc. reduce the fire and increase the burden on the digestive system. **Please note that Heat is Life while Cold is Death. Eat or drink accordingly.**

**Sprouted Pulses :** The beans like green peas and gram (चना) etc. which can be splited into exact two parts should be first sprouted and may be taken by all people uncooked, but can be mixed while preparing green juice or mixed with til (sesame), groundnut, raw cabbage, dates, dried grapes or a little jaggery. They have vitamin B Complex, plenty of vitamins C and E, proteins and minerals. Children, expectant mothers and old people should be given this important food. Sprouted pulses are also very good for reducing weight. In that case the use of dates, dried grapes or jaggery should be avoided.

**Test of proper digestive power and proper eating :** After the meals, you should feel energetic, light in body and capable of work – even running if necessary. If you feel heavy, sleepy or dull, it indicates overeating or fast eating or a weakened digestive system.

**Assistance of Acupressure for the digestive system :** Sit on a chair. Keep the wooden roller on the ground, giving as much pressure as possible, roll the feet on the foot roller for five minutes-each foot. This will activate all the organs of the digestive system, kidney, lungs, etc. It is of great help to people above the age of 40 *(See fig. 69)*. They should increase the use of ginger, *Amla* and lemon in their diet.

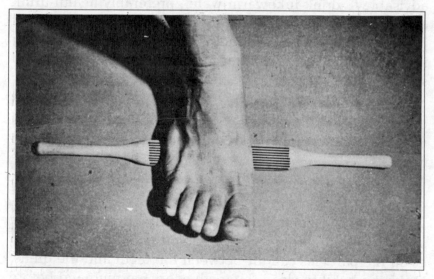

Fig. 69

**Laxatives :** Laxatives are not necessary. Check up the Solar Plexus and correct it if necessary. Give pressure or rub on the middle of the chin for 3 to 6 minutes in the morning or while in W. C. to ensure the cleaning of the bowels and thus avoid constipation which is the root cause of many diseases *(See fig. 111)*. For a long term cure of constipation.

( 1 ) Drink two to three glasses of lukewarm or hot water first thing in the morning. Lie on your back and roll the wooden roller on the stomach / abdomen.

( 2 ) Drink 6 to 8 glasses of water during the day. If possible, drink buttermilk twice daily.

( 3 ) Include leafy vegetables in your diet.

( 4 ) Chew properly and roll your feet on a grooved wooden roller, 5 minutes every evening to increase your digestive power.

**Stools :** Occasionally observe the stools . Nature gives us good indication of our digestive system. Odourless, properly formed dry stools floating in water or easily cleansible, indicate proper digestion. Otherwise, it is advisable to drink lukewarm water, preferably health drink or copper / silver / gold charged water, (Method of preparation has been described in Chapter 14) the first thing in the morning and take light food avoiding fried items and sweets.

**How to correct Digestive power :** In case of long term complaint about the disorders of the stomach, digestion, biles etc, it is found useful to take the following medicine for 4 to 6 weeks.

Nux Vomica 200×4 Pills twice a week.⎫(a Homeopathic
Nux Vomica 12×4 Pills twice daily.   ⎭ medicine)

**Dental Care and Mouth Care :** After every meal, chew a little salt and gargle with water. Soft brush can be used to clean the particles caught between the teeth and the gums. Make it a habit to clean the teeth every morning and before retiring to bed. In India, people use thin twig of a Babul, Banyan or a Neem tree (known as Datoon) as a brush. First it is to be crushed to make it soft and then use it like a brush. It is advisable to use a Datoon of Babul, Banyan or Neem tree at least once a day.

It is reported by experienced dentists that tooth pastes available in the market are not much effective. Instead, the following tooth powder or paste which can be easily made at home has been found quite useful for the care of gums and teeth :

**( 1 ) Tooth Powder :** Mixture of finely ground alum powder 40% and rock salt or regular salt powder 60%. For better results, a few drops of lemon may be added. In case of dental problems, adding a little of 'Sudarshan' (a bitter Ayurvedic powder) is also recommended.

**( 2 ) Tooth-paste :** For dental problems like bleeding, pyorrhoea, toothache, etc. make a paste of

50% alum powder

10% rock salt or table salt powder

10% Sudarshan powder (an Ayurvedic preparation)

15% edible oil (unrefined)

10% glycerine tanic acid

5% camphor.

The paste made of this mixture can be massaged on the teeth and gums in the morning and evening with fingers. It can be packed in collapsible tubes/jars and used as tooth-paste.

**( 3 ) Even massaging the gums** with a mixture of 70% unrefined edible oil (seasame or groundnut or coconut), 15% glycerine tanic acid and 15% fine powder of rock salt or table salt is useful for good, healthy teeth and gums. Make it a daily habit. Please note that healthy gums are more useful than sparkling white teeth.

**( 4 ) Mouth Freshener :** Gargling with a little lemon juice mixed with lukewarm water, freshens the mouth. Take a quarter of a lemon, massage it on teeth and gums and then gargle with water. Even chewing of mango, tulsi or betel leaves after meals is good, and so it is advised in India.

**( 5 ) Exercises for teeth :** Keep the lips closed. Pound the upper teeth on lower teeth for 30 to 40 times twice a day. Then massage the saliva on gums with the tongue. That will ensure proper blood circulation in teeth and increase the life of healthy teeth and gums.

**( 6 ) Tongue :** It is necessary that the tongue is cleaned properly with a metallic or non-metallic tongue cleaner. This will clear the congestion not only on the tongue but also of the throat. Moreover, as all the meridians pass through the tongue, little massaging of the tongue with a tongue cleaner, will activate all the organs below the diaphragm. The use of the tongue cleaner is recommended three times daily especially in case of tonsils, congestion in the throat, diphtheria, etc. Now, cleaning of the tongue is accepted in the U.S.A.

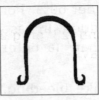

**Tongue Cleaner**

**Skin Care :** The Skin is porous and throws out toxins from the body. So it is very necessary to maintain its health. For the care of the skin it is necessary to :

( 1 ) drink plenty of water (6 to 8 glasses), if possible health drink 3 to 4 times a day.

( 2 ) eat groundnuts, til (sesame) or any type of nuts especially in winter and plenty of seasonal vegetables and fruits.

( 3 ) have oil massage once a week or at least twice a month.

( 4 ) take sunbath early in the morning regularly.

( 5 ) practise Pranayam regularly.

( 6 ) avoid eating foodstuffs in such combination as would create disturbance/toxins in the body/blood. For example,

| Avoid eating any one of the following : | with any one of the following : |
|---|---|
| Pulses<br>Garlic, Onion, Fish,<br>Antibiotics<br>Citrus fruits | Milk (unwarmed up)<br>Buttermilk/curd or<br>Milk preparation |

( 7 ) Drink daily 2 to 3 cups of green juice.

( 8 ) Apply waste of green juice paste adding in it little turmeric powder and cream of milk on all affected parts; also on the face as face mask then take a blue light for 6 to 8 minutes on it and wash with water and observe the astonishing results in 15/20 days.

( 9 ) Also activate the points No. 22 and 23 of gall bladder and liver if necessary three times a day.

(10) When the skin becomes dry and there is a lot of itching, on the affected parts, apply/massage coconut oil which is to be prepared as under :

Put garlic in a little quantity of cocount oil and boil it. Let it cool down. Then filter it and keep it in a bottle. This oil can also be used as ear drops too.

**Posture :** It is observed that most people complaining about digestive problems, backache and pain in the legs, do not usually sit in an upright, straight position, especially when sitting on the ground. Upright posture is a must for good health. By stooping, the stomach and abdomen are not allowed to expand properly while breathing and that puts extra pressure on the lungs. Moreover, the spinal column is damaged. See figure 20 and 22.

The result is an improper functioning of the stomach, abdomen and sciatic nerve leading to less oxygenation. The first thing is to change the way of sitting. One must sit upright. Secondly, when seated on a chair with back upright, take out the breath and then pull in and expand the stomach and abdomen. Do this for 8 to 10 minutes a day. This is a good exercise for all especially to avoid gas, indigestion, fat, etc. But this must be done either before meals or at least two hours after meals.

**Test of good health :**
( 1 ) The head should be cool.
( 2 ) The soles should be warm.
( 3 ) The stomach should be soft, which is possible only if constipation is avoided and solar plexus is in order.

Now in case the head is warmer, and the soles cooler, as is in case of cold due to heat, Meningitis, brain's problems, Parkinson's disease, Arthritis, Stroke, chronic disease, etc. do the following :

Take a nylon brush which is used for washing the clothes. Rub it under the soles for 3 to 5 minutes three times a day till the soles become warmer.

**Germs :** The germs of disease enter our body (a) through water and/or the drink we take and/or (b) through the food we eat. Wherever (1) purified water is not available, water should be boiled as is done by the Jains in India and by most people in China, (2) when we eat food, proper care should be taken not to eat–

( 1 ) fruits or eatables kept in the open without washing.

( 2 ) overripe and spoiled fruits

( 3 ) diseased fish or polluted meat of diseased animals.

If the above suggestions are followed properly, causes of diseases are reduced to a great extent. And the minor ailments due to change of weather, water and food can be controlled with Acupressure treatment. The net result will be good health throughout life.

# CHAPTER 6

# NATURE CURE

Nature cure means following the rules of Nature and curing the disease with the help of the elements of Nature viz. earth, water, sun and air, in such a way that toxins collected in the body are thrown out so that body becomes pure and life current powerful. This enables the body to cure the diseases and make the body work efficiently.

**Earth / Mud :** Due to the rising problems of germs in the earth, the placing of wet mud pack on the stomach and other affected parts is less advocated. However, the paste of green juice can be applied. Such a pack can be put on the eyes, stomach and skin . When it becomes dry, green juice can be sprinkled on it or the green pack can be changed. For better results, after applying green pack, sunrays or Blue light can be taken on it. The results are wonderful even in case of white spots (leukoderma / leprosy.)

**Water :** ( 1 ) Drink plenty of water 8 to 10 glasses every day. In India, there was a custom of drinking 2 to 3 glasses of water kept overnight in a copper vessel and then walk for about one mile before going to the toilet in the open. Recently, a Japanese professor tried this method on 30,000 people and was convinced of the great benefits of drinking first thing in the morning, 2 to 3 glasses of water boiled the previous night and kept in a metal vessel.

**Drinking water in the morning :** Keep boiled water in a metal vessel preferably copper overnight. In the morning even without cleaning the teeth or gargling, drink 3 to 5 glasses of this water. You can begin with 1 to 2 glasses. Increase the quantity to 4 to 5 glasses of water i.e 1 litre to $1\frac{1}{2}$ litres. Then walk for 10/15 minutes. If walking is not possible, lie down on back and roll wooden roller on the stomach. This practice will remove not only constipation but also excess heat from the body and many diseases connected with excess heat. Before drinking water in the morning, check up the Solar Plexus and correct it if necessary. During the day also drink plenty of water–8 to 10 glasses of water.

The habit of drinking water in the morning plus doing Acupressure regularly will greatly minimise the possibility of diseases.

( 2 ) Use of hot and cold pack is shown on page 200 of this book. Application of cold pack helps in reducing fever and removing the morbid matter (toxin) from the body. Hot pack on the other hand relieves pain and swelling.

( 3 ) Vapour treatment and steam bath are useful to drive out the cold and toxins from the affected part through perspiration and increased circulation of blood. It is very useful in polio, arthritis, rheumatism, paralysis, etc.

( 4 ) Moreover, if facilities are available, one can take hip bath in a tub filled with cold and hot water. The level of water should be upto the navel.

( 5 ) In case of fever, wet cotton bedsheet can be wrapped over the body and covered with woollen blanket for 15 to 30 minutes. This can be repeated after 1 to 2 hours if necessary.

**Air :** Pure air is a great doctor. Methods of easy Pranayams are, therefore shown in this book on page 111/113. If Mudras, shown on page are also carried out at the same time, better and faster results can be obtained.

**Sun :** As it is of utmost importance a special chapter No. 7 is devoted to it in this book.

**Diet :** As mentioned in chapter 2, natural products like vegetables, fruits, sprouted pulses have equal quantity of positive and negative sun energy stored in them. Therefore, they are easily digested and they give the maximum energy.

**Fasting :** In order to remove the toxins mostly in the digestive organs, fasting of 24 to 72 hours or more is advocated. During fasting it is advisable to drink lukewarm boiled water and green juices. One can make it a practice to skip a meal once a week. Skip meals for a day once a month and remain on boiled water, green juices and fruit juices for three days in a year. Such fasts should be broken with fruit juices.

**Body and its electricity :** The best element of Nature is our body (its bio-energy) and one can easily use it oneself through. Acupressure which has been narrated in this book at length.

One should not forget that even an advanced and best, man is also an animal of Nature and therefore more and more use of these basic elements of nature will give good health. For faster and guaranteed results, use of these therapies of nature to the maximum extent should be made simultaneously.

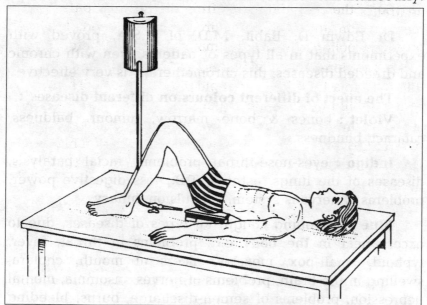

Fig. 70 : How to take enema

**Enema :** In order to remove stools from big intestines, enema should be taken with lukewarm water. One teaspoon of coffee powder and one teaspoon of castor oil can be added to the water for better results. Even 50% healthy self urine can be added in 50% water. During and after the fast, enema is very useful. Such enema should be followed with enema of cold water.

# CHAPTER 7

# CHROMOTHERAPY–USE OF COLOURS OF THE SUN

In the Vedas, the sun is greatly praised and rightly so. Our cosmos exists because of the sun. All the living beings get their energy from the sun. And this energy is abundant and unlimited, so it should be used to the maximum.

The sun looks white, but it consists of seven colours viz. violet, indigo, blue, green, yellow, orange and red. Out of these the first three have cool effect on the body and are also antiseptic. The last three colours create heat. Green is neutral.

Dr Edwin D. Babit, M.D. of U.S.A. proved with experiments that in all types of patients even with chronic and dreaded diseases, this chromotherapy is very effective.

**The effect of different colours on different diseases :**

**Violet :** bones & bone marrow, tumour, baldness, cataract, blindness.

**Indigo :** eyes-nose-throat problems, facial paralysis, diseases of the lungs, asthma, T.B., less digestive power, problems of nervous system, convulsion, lunacy.

**Blue :** whooping cough, all types of diseases, due to excess heat in the body e.g. problems in throat, fever, typhoid, small-pox, measles, ulcers in mouth, cholera, swelling in the brain, problems of nerves, insomnia, mental depression, problems of semen-discharge, burns, bleeding from nose, etc.

Dr Edwin Babit calls the blue colour as the world's best antiseptic and that is why the cloudless blue sky during the day has great beneficial influence on the world.

**Green :** heart problems, low & high B.P., skin problems, cancer, influenza, syphilis, pain in the eyes, etc.

**Yellow :** All disorders of digestion, spleen, liver problems, diabetes, leprosy, etc.

**Orange :** longterm asthma, bronchitis, swelling in trachea, gout, swelling, kidney, mental-nervousness, epilepsy, etc.

**Red :** anaemia, disability, sluggishness, cold, paralysis, white spots, arthritis., T.B., etc.

**How to take rays :** 90 minutes from sunrise and 60 minutes before sunset; keep a glass of desired colour in the sunlight in such a way that the rays will fall on the affected parts. While taking sunlight care should be taken to see that the patient is not exposed to strong direct wind.

If that is not possible, take a coloured bulb of 60 to 100 watts. If such a coloured bulb is not available, take a plain bulb, take coloured gelatin paper, fourfold the same and wrap it around the bulb, light the lamp, keep the affected part 18 to 20 inches away and take the light for 5 to 10 minutes twice a day.

**How to take colours through water :** Take a glass bottle of the desired colour. If it is not available, wrap gelatin paper of the desired colour on the white glass bottle. Fill it 3/4th and keep it on a wooden plank. And keep it in sunlight for at least 3 hours between 10 a.m. and 3 p.m. Even if such a bottle is kept in the sunlight for more than 3 hours, it is not harmful. Just take care that this type of coloured water is not exposed to any other type of colour.

Now, half a glass colour medicated water can be given to the patient at an interval of 15 to 20 minutes depending upon the intensity of the disease. In case, the water of other colours is necessary, it can be given alternatively.

This is the therapy of Nature and can be effectively used with Acupressure. An Acupressurist should study this therapy and use it with care.

---

# CHAPTER 8

# URINE THERAPY

Even the allopathic doctors in the west, have accepted that to fight and clear toxins from the body, our own body creates antibodies. Now, during sleep the computer of our body manufactures such medicine according to specific requirements of the individual and is present in a big quantity in the first urine in the morning. And so, if the first urine is drunk, the body will get all its requirements, salts, etc. This is the principle of this therapy. Realising its great medicinal value, costly life saving injections are prepared from urine in Japan.

It may be surprising to note that even in the religious scriptures like Shivpuran, Mahabharat, Bible, etc., it is mentioned that **this urine is the nectar of life** and details about how to drink the same are very well narrated in Shivpuran. Even the culprits know the benefit of the urine. Whenever they are caught, the first thing they do, is to drink their own urine, so that when they get a heavy beating, they can recover from it very soon. Even in long fasting, it is advised to drink one's urine.

Sri Morarjibhai Desai, the former Prime Minister of India and a great propagator of this Urine therapy, used to drink his urine and massage the same on his body for 40 years till his death at the age of 100. That was the secret of his reddishness till the last minute. His skin was healthy and had no wrinkles. It was smooth and glowing.

At the age of 61, cataract started in his eyes. He started using his urine as eye-wash and cured his cataract and had no need to get cataract removed till the age of 91 – thus he prevented cataract formation for 30 years.

In all types of chronic diseases, it is advisable to drink one's urine. Dr Beatrice Barter of U.S.A claims to have cured even patients of AIDS with urine therapy. I am of the opinion, that if treatment mentioned in this book for cancer of blood and thalasemmia is combined with this urine therapy, the problem of AIDS can be controlled quite easily and rapidly.

**How to Use :** Let the first few drops pass. Then collect the urine in a clean glass / tumbler or in hands and drink it.

**For Eyes :** Keep it in an eye glass or in the palm and use it as an eye wash after the urine has cooled down. It is effective to keep eyes in good condition and to cure the beginning of cataract.

**Teeth :** For any types of problems of teeth – even when teeth are shaking, gargle this urine for at least five minutes. Massage it on the gums.

**Care of Hair :** Massaging of urine on hair and scalp makes the hair soft and silky, clears dandruff, germs, etc. It can be applied on the face before a shave as a shaving cream and it will give a clean smooth shave and afterwards can also be used as after shave lotion. Such an application enhances the glow of face, and so can be very well used by both men and women. It will be found to be one of the best shampoos.

**Skin Problems :** It is one of the best medicines for the skin. In the book, the use of urine in syphilis, gangrene, white spots, etc. has been separately explained.

**How to Apply on Skin :** Warm the first urine, let it cool down. The crust has to be removed. Soak cotton in this lukewarm urine and massage it on affected parts for 2 to 5 minutes. Before doing so, massage ice on the affected parts for 2 to 3 minutes. Afterwards, wash with clean water.

At the same if two to three cups of green juice is drunk daily and colour treatment is taken the results are astounding; it even cures white spots.

**Precaution :** Before using self urine, please get it 'Tested'. It should not contain **'Sugar'** or **'Pus'. If it contains sugar or pus, take the treatment to cure the same, and do not use your urine till then.**

# CHAPTER 9

# TWELVE SALTS-BIOCHEMIC THERAPY

The water in our body and the water of sea are the same. The water we drink does not contain the salts of sea water or those in our body. We get the necessary salts from the vegetables and other food. Sometimes, if we are not able to take enough quantity of such salts, there would be a deficiency of such salt in our body which in turn can create diseases in the body. And when we take such salts as medicines the diseases are cured. Dr Shusler of Germany has made a research about the same known as Biochemistry. He has maintained that there are billions of tiny cells in the body and so if any of these twelve salts is taken in such tiny form, it will reach these cells of our body and cure it and make it work properly.

Now, from experience it has been observed that these salts should be given on the first day of the week in the potency (power) of 200 and in 12 or 30 for the rest six days. Continue such treatment for four to six weeks as may be necessary.

This is an innocent therapy.The patient can take it himself. If necessary more than one salt can be combined and taken together. It is very useful for children.

These medicines supplement the Acupressure treatment and so in this book these medicines are prescribed. An Acupressurist should, if possible, acquire proper knowledge about these biochemic medicines.

Here in the following table you will find the names of these twelve biochemic salts (medicines), where the place of such salts is in the body and for which diseases they are useful.

| Name | Place | Useful in Which Disease |
| --- | --- | --- |
| 1. Calcar, Phos (Calcium Phosphate) | Teeth, Bones, Blood & Tissues | Useful for all problems connected with teeth, bones, blood & tissues, in all problems connected with tissues i. e. worry, cold, less appetite. breathing, painful urination, etc. |
| 2. Calcar Sulf (Calcium Sulphate) | Lying between the tissues. | Useful for–driving out toxins, cold, coughing, T.B., boils, ulcer, swelling in ears, pus & blood in urine, arthritis, etc. |
| 3. Cal. Flour (Calcium Floride) | Nerves, Muscles | It gives contraction, So where-ever these nerves and muscles have become loose, this medicine is used to give them tone. |
| 4. Ferrum Phos (Ferrous phosphate) | in the blood cells. | Anaemia, all problems due to deficiency in blood, all types of fever, lack of concentration, forgetfulness. |
| 5. Kali Muir (Pottassium Chloride) | Blood muscles & Nerves | For all problems regarding blood-nerves, indigestion, vomi-ting–loose motions, and in swelling of delicate nerves, good for all breathing problems. |
| 6. Kali Phosv (Potassium Phosphate) | Brain–nerves & muscles | All the problems connected with brain & central nervous system– is considered king of all twelve salts. |
| 7. Kali sulf (Potassium sulphate) | Skin & arteries | All problems of skin due to improper functioning of perspi-ration or due to germs, arthritis-fever. Useful to ladies to increase skin beauty. |

| Name | Place | Useful in Which Disease |
|------|-------|-------------------------|
| 8. Mag. Phos (Magnesium phosphate) | Muscles, bone marrow | It is expanding vasodilator, all types of pains headaches convulsions. epilepsy and paralysis, etc. |
| 9. Natrum Muir (Sodium chloride) | Water of the body | Sunstroke, dehydration, Insomnia – weakness of brain – palpitation, etc. |
| 10. Natrum Phos. (Sodium Phosphate) | Water of Body | Acidity, worms, dullness of memory, improper functioning of the heart. |
| 11. Natrum Sulph (Sodium Sulphate) | Water of Body | Controls water in the body, produces more urine: |
| 12. Silica | Water of Body | This is the element of earth-works as a surgeon of body, very useful in boils. |

Further it has been observed with in depth research that zodiac signs play an important part on the basic deficiency of certain salts in the body and which in turn, lead to certain problems (diseases) as mentioned above. Moreover, certain salts are found to be supplementary. So, a chart is given below of combinations of such basic salts (which are useful to all the persons – children and adults of all ages) and the corresponding zodiac signs with birth dates.

| Combination of Biochemic Medicines : | Effective on Zodiac Signs of | Birthdates |
|---------------------------------------|------------------------------|------------|
| 1. Kali Phos | Aries | 22 – 3 to 21 – 4 |
| Cal. Fl. | Cancer | 22 – 6 to 21 – 7 |
| Cal. Phos. | Libra | 22 – 9 to 21 – 10 |
| Nat. Phos. | Capricorn | 22 – 12 to 21 – 1 |
| Fer. Phos. | | |

2. Nat. Sulph ⎫ Taurus 22−4 to 21−5
   Cal. Sulph ⎪ Leo 22−7 to 21−8
   Mag. Phos ⎬ Scorpio 22−10 to 21−11
   Nat. Mur ⎪ Aquarius 22−1 to 21−2
   Kali Phos ⎭

3. Kali Muir ⎫ Pieces 22−2 to 21−3
   Kali Sulph ⎪ Gemini 22−5 to 21−6
   Silicia ⎬ Virgo 22−8 to 21−9
   Fer. Phos ⎪ Sagittarius 22−11 to 21−12
   Kali Phos ⎭

**Method :**

Make a combination of 6x     1oz
Make a combination of 12x     1oz
Make a combination of 200     1/2 oz
combination of 200 to be taken once a week.
combination of 6x to be taken for 4 weeks.
Then no medicine to be taken for two weeks.
Then
combination of 200 to be taken once a week.
combination of 12x to be taken for 4 weeks.

After every one year, repeat as above for 2 weeks with 6x, no medicine for a week and then 2 weeks with 12x and during all that time 200 once a week.

| Dose | Morning | Afternoon | Evening |
|---|---|---|---|
| Children under 5 | 2 | 2 | 2 pills |
| Children under 15 | 3 | 3 | 3 pills |
| For all over 15 | 4 | 4 | 4 pills |

Now, if allopathic medicines are being given previously, in order to nullify its effects; first give one dose of 4 pills Thuja 200 once in a day for 3 days only.

This supplementation of basic salts can be done by all people of any age group.

Moreover these biochemic medicines can be put in a glass bottle of desired colour for 3 to 5 hours in the sun to get faster relief.

In this way, if these bio-chemic medicines (basic salts) are taken, alongwith regular treatment of Acupressure, the possibility of diseases will be reduced to the minimum.

———

# CHAPTER 10

# CHILD CARE

Children are like the flowers of the Garden-that is-this world, and we all would like them to blossom fully. Children are closer to God, and so their divine laughter is always enchanting. It is no wonder then that Mahatma Gandhi and Pandit Jawaharlal Nehru saw the image of God in them.

If we want to stop wars and unnecessary killings on this planet, we must all start taking care of children not only of their physical health but also of their mental health and make sure that when they grow up, they have a healthy and happy approach towards life.

The care of children's health does not start only after their birth. Even before the baby is conceived in the mother's womb, both the parents must take care to see to it that they themselves are in proper healthy condition of mind and body so that the child to be born does not inherit any disease of the mind or body.

**Planning of Children :**

This can be considered in three parts : (1) Before conception, (2) During conception and (3) After conception.

( 1 ) (a) Parenthood should be properly planned and should not be a matter of accident. It has been found by the western people that oral contraceptives have harmful side-effects and so are no longer recommended.

(b) The couple must start the treatment under Acupressure therapy at least 3 months prior to conceiving, to ensure their proper health, creation of hormones and curing of any possible disease that they themselves suffer from.

(c) The couple should drink one glass each of gold/silver/copper/iron charged water (4 glasses reduced to 2 glasses) per day.

(d) The wife must have 5 to 7 regular menses before conceiving.

The total effect of the above would be to get a fully developed, healthy, child with the possibility of inheriting hereditary problems reduced to the minimum. **Even those couples desiring children but not getting them would get their desire fulfilled if they take treatment, especially on both the sides of the two wrists for 4 to 6 minutes** (Pressure Points No. 11 to 15), daily alongwith the treatment mentioned above.

**( 2 ) How to get the child of the desired sex :** Please refer to page no. 114 about Pranayam. It is claimed by Ayurved that the following methods, if followed by the couple, will give them the child of the desired sex.

(a) The day on which the menses are seen, is to be counted as the first day.

(b) During the period of flow, the couple should strictly avoid intercourse. For guaranteed results, intercourse is to be done only once in a month on any one of the dates mentioned below. Continue the plan till baby is conceived.

( c ) **For getting a son :** On the even dates, i. e. 4th, 6th, 8th, 10th, 12th, or 14th day, the husband should lie with his wife on his left side for 15 minutes so that he would be breathing with his right nostril before the intercourse.

(d) **For getting a daughter :** On the odd dates i. e. 5th, 7th, 9th, 11th, 13th or 15th day, the husband should lie with his wife on his right side for 15 minutes so that he would be breathing with his left nostril before the intercourse.

It has also been advised in Ayurved that if the intercourse is done during the later dates (10th to 15th) there is a greater possibility of conceiving and the child to be born will be healthier.

**( 3 )** (a) After the baby is conceived, the mother should take proper care about its nourishment. She should eat plenty of seasonal fruits. In order to get natural calcium, she should drink more milk and eat bananas. Otherwise she should take daily 4 pills in morning and 4 pills in the evening of Cal. phos 12x + Cal. Fl. 12x (mixed together – Biochemic medicines) for calcium. If sufficient calcium is taken throughout the pregnancy and proper diet is taken by the mother, the child to be born will not have any problem of teeth and bone development later on. According to the research work done in China, it has been found out that if properly controlled diet is taken by the mother during pregnancy, the child will have less craving for sweet things like chocolates, biscuits, etc.

Now, if the newly born child is not given sweets for twelve months, then according to American Dentist Association, the possibility of having a dental problem in child's life will be reduced.

(b) The expectant mother should practise the Acu-pressure therapy daily to ensure good health and freedom from disease and to reduce the possibility of miscarriage. Atleast give pressure treatment on the two sides of the wrists to prevent miscarriage. (Point No. 11 to 15)

(c) The expectant mother should drink iron/copper/silver and gold charged water, two glasses reduced from four glasses. This will ensure the birth of a healthy baby and reduce the possibility of the baby being blind and that of retardedness or muscular distrophy, etc. after its birth.

(d) The expectant mother should do some light exercise daily at least walking 2 to 3 kilometres.

(e) **The child starts learning while in the mother's womb,** The cases of Abhimanyu and Shukdev are very famous. So the expectant mother must try to be cheerful, read and listen to books on religion, art, music and culture, etc.

(f) The husband should also help the wife in all these activities and keep her cheerful during this vital period of pregnancy.

**Care after the birth of a baby :** The birth of a healthy child solves many a problem. With proper nourishment and rest, the child will grow normally. Further, if Acupressure treatment is given on the soles of the baby every day only for 3 to 4 minutes, good development will be ensured and there won't be any major problem of health.

We must not forget that the children are very close to Nature and the requirements for a good crop. viz., good seed, enough manure, water and light are also essential for children's growth. They require proper nourishing diet, mother's loving care and play which includes sunshine and rest.

*Mrs. 'L' reports that her three months old grandson had complaints of vomitting milk and retarded progress and often cried. With regular massage on the soles, the child grows happily without giving any trouble.*

**Care and treatment of children from the age of 1 day to 14 years :**

( 1 ) After the baby is born, it should be breast-fed at least for 9 to 12 months and during that time the mother should take care of her diet, eat proper nourishing food and drink iron/copper/silver/gold charged water. If nothing else is possible, take hot meals twice a day. She should also practise Acupressure therapy to prevent any disease and tension. If milk other than mother's (preferably goat's or camel's only, otherwise cow's milk) is to be given, please add a little water to it. (preferably iron/copper/silver/gold charged)

( 2 ) Between 7 – 9 months, at the time of teething, care should be taken to supplement the diet of the child with calcium. If it is not possible to give bananas and more milk, the child may be given Calcaria Phos + Cal. Fl 6x or 12x – two pills of each twice a day.

( 3 ) Proper attention should be paid to cleanliness and hygiene. Change the nappies, diapers, etc., every time the child urinates or passes stools and clean the parts with wet cloth. Wash the child's clothes daily and sterilise them at least once in 3 days by boiling them or by keeping them for some time in water containing antiseptics like Dettol and then wash them.

( 4 ) **Sleep :** This is most vital to children of every age especially upto 12 months. If the child gets proper sleep alongwith proper nourishment, half the battle against diseases is won.

( 5 ) **Water :** Most of the infections come through water, so please be careful to give boiled water to the child. It is necessary that schools should arrange to provide boiled water duly cooled and filtered to the children.

( 6 ) **Bath and Soap :** Give the baby a bath with lukewarm water after an oil massage. Use soap most sparingly. Instead, paste made of cream of milk and gram flour should be used. Please note that by using soap in excess you are harming the tender skin of the baby. Moreover, the use of soap will not make the skin any fairer.

( 7 ) **Air and Sun :** Just as in the growth of plants and animals, air and sun play an important role in the development of the human body also. When the child completes 3 months, after an oil massage, put the child in the sun for at least 10/15 minutes after 90 minutes of sunrise. Please see that the child is taken out daily to get fresh air. After the baby learns to stand on its legs, let him/her play out of the house during the day for at least 45/60 minutes.

Food, rest and play are the most vital factors for the proper development of the body and the mind of the child.

( 8 ) **Sugar :** In modern times, the use of sugar has increased greatly. Avoid it as far as possible, at least till the baby is 12 months old. Afterwards, sugar may be used. Instead of white sugar, use crystal sugar or jaggery. Please see that it is added to milk or water at the time of boiling. Do not add sugar afterwards. This will help in preventing cold and cough.

**( 9 ) Cold drinks, ice-creams and chocolates :** In spite of many warnings, parents and children still indulge in these foods. To counter the adverse effects of these harmful foods, the best way is to give lukewarm water to the child at least 2/3 times a day. Give them bitter powder like 'Sudarshan' which will prevent worms and enhance digestive power.

**(10) The child's motion :** Regular motions and clear urination are most vital. In the case of loose motion or unsatisfactory motions, the best course is to stop milk or food intake. And try to put the child on lukewater and juice of vegetables and fruits at least for a meal or two. That will automatically help the body to get over the troubles.

In boiling milk, put a few drops of lemon juice, water will get separated from paneer, If necessary, add a little sugar and lemon drops and only give this separated water to drink. The paneer can be used for preparing vegetables.

Please note that no child will die if kept hungry for half a day or even a day Overfeeding disturbs the whole digestive system and leads to many diseases.

**(11) Treatment :** It is most vital and important that treatment of Acupressure therapy is given daily for 3 to 4 minutes on each palm and/or on the soles. This will definitely prevent the possibility of disease and ensure the progress of the children in body, mind and character.

After the child has completed 8 years, 4 to 5 minutes treatment on each palm should be given daily and he/she should be taught to continue the same life long.

While giving the treatment, the child will immediately cry if there is any pain due to pressure on any point. This gives a clue to the disease, which can be easily cured by this treatment.

If proper nourishment is given to children as per the table given below, along with proper care as mentioned earlier, most of the children will not suffer from any serious disease.

**Diet for Child :**

**1 day to 3 months old :** Milk (breast-feeding) otherwise goat's, camel's milk or cow's milk.

**4 Months to 9 months :** Milk (breast-feeding) goat's, camel's or cow's milk plus seasonal fruit juice plus mashed rice and banana.

**10 months to 15 months :** Goat's, camel's or cow's milk plus fruits-bananas are a must, plus mashed rice/khichdi and potatoes, chapatis/whole wheat bread, etc., when the child can chew.

**16 months to 15 years :** Milk plus food containing protein like wheat, sprouted pulses like mung. Chinese green Peas, grams, etc., all types of nuts plus seasonal fruits.

**(12)** Supplement the deficiency of birth salts as shown in chapter 9 of this book.

As the children are not able to tell about their problem, this therapy is most useful in immediate and proper diagnosis. Along with this treatment, Biochemic medicines can be added to get quick, amazing results.

Just for a petty symptom, do not get panicky. Take the treatment of Acupressure therapy, reduce the quantity of milk or food and give more of lukewarm water, fruit juice and fruits and within 48 hours the child will be normal, laughing to its heart's content.

**Special Instructions for mothers :**

( 1 ) Right from 1st day, press daily each sole of your sweet child for 2 to 3 minutes till your baby becomes 1 year old.

( 2 ) Then press daily 3 to 4 minutes in each palm or sole-till 8 th birthday.

( 3 ) Then daily teach her / him how to press each palm for 4 to 5 minutes.

( 4 ) Give your child daily 2 to 3 teaspoonsrf charged water till 60 days. If he / she gets reddishness in stool, reduce the quantum of gold.

From 61 days to 2 years give a $\frac{1}{4}$ galss of charged water to drink. Then 2 years to 5 years $\frac{1}{2}$ glass. From 5 years to 10 years 1 glass. Wherever possible, give this water lukewarm.

(5) Every six months, check about worms and if necessary, give treatment for same.

(6) Checkup solar plexus every alternate day and if necessary correct it.

(7) After 4 months, start giving $\frac{1}{4}$ cup of green juice and after 1 year give $\frac{1}{2}$ cup to 1 cup adding $\frac{1}{4}$ tsp health powder and $\frac{1}{4}$ tsp honey.

(8) At least once in 15 days, skip one feeding, give warm water/green juice.

(9) Every week give mild laxative like harde.

---

# CHAPTER 11

# WOMEN'S PROBLEMS

Woman is different from man as regards sex and temperament. Moreover, Nature has given her an additional responsibility of becoming a mother. She has to pay special attention not only to maintain good health but also to remain calm and happy. She also needs proper education on childcare and household duties. She will be capable of handling all these responsibilities properly, if she is healthy. **It would greatly benefit women to learn about Acupressure. Regular Acupressure treatment will help them to prevent nervous tension and breakdown, hysteria, timidness, frigidity, etc. It is advisable for them to take the treatment shown for nervous tension and on all the endocrine glands from an early age of 6 – 7 years onwards. This will also save them from the problems of menses and ensure healthy growth of their body and mind.**

( 1 ) **Problems of Menses :** In problems of menstruation. namely early, irregular or painful menstruation, scanty or excessive bleeding or backache, before, during or after menses, etc. treatment of points No. 11 to 15 and on all points of endocrine glands will show amazing results. Such treatment can be taken by massaging these points on the two sides of the wrists.

If this treatment is continued menstruation will be regular within 2 to 3 months and all the problems connected with it will be solved.

*Dr 'K' reports that Miss 'T' had the problem of scanty and painful menstruation while Mrs. 'Y' had excessive bleeding. In both the cases treatment was given on points No. 11 to 15 and the patients were cured effectively. There were no complaints afterwards. A number of similar cases have been treated successfully by Acupressure therapy.*

( 2 ) **Profuse Bleeding :** In case of excessive bleeding, rubber bands may be applied on the base of both the big toes for 3/5 minutes and this may be repeated after 15/20 minutes, if necessary (Fig. 71).

( 3 ) **Leucorrhoea :**
For leucorrhoea also,
treatment on Points No.
11 to 15 will be useful. It
is also advisable to drink
g o l d / s i l v e r / c o p p e r
charged water (1 glass
reduced from 2 glasses).
Moreover, take the
treatment of Anaemia as
mentioned below. Also
sit on a ball for 5 to 10
minutes twice a day as
shown in fig. 80.

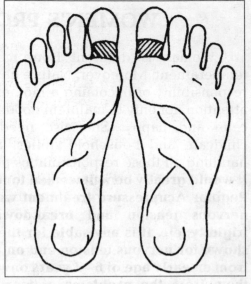

Fig. 71

*Mrs. 'Y' was*
*suffering from leucor-*
*rhoea for the past*
*seven years and had tried many medicines without success.*
*After just 3 sittings of Acupressure treatment, 70% of her*
*complaints had gone and within 20 days of this treatment she*
*was free from the dreaded disease.*

( 4 ) **Menopause :** For ladies over 40 years, this problem
can start especially in the case of those who are less active
and rather more sentimental and care more for the family.

With regular treatment on all points especially
No. 11 to 15 and all endocrine glands and treatment for
nervous tension, this problem can be solved easily. Even the
period of menses will be prolonged. There will be more
interest and joy in married life and the diseases connected
with this period will be easily overcome. After the age of 40,
all the women should make this treatment their daily routine.
Further, treatment on these points will save women from
timidness and frigitidy.

( 5 ) **Planning    forchildren :** Before    planning    for
children, it is essential for the couple to have this treatment
for at least 3 to 4 months before conceiving the child in order
to prevent any hereditary disease. For those couples not
getting children, such treatment for 4 to 6 months, taken by
both, greatly enhances the chances of conceiving.

**( 6 ) Prevention of Miscarriage :** After the child is conceived, it is essential to take this treatment regularly to **prevent miscarriage** and to reduce the possibility of any diseases. It will also ensure proper growth of the child to be born.

**( 7 ) Painless Childbirth :** At the time of the first delivery, the mother is very much worried and is under great tension. This adds to the labour pains. Sometimes, it has been observed that owing to greater pain or delayed delivery, the child is vitally affected not only in body but also in mind. Even in the case of the use of forceps or caesarean operation, the child's body may get damaged and even the mother may be hurt. It is, therefore, essential that the delivery is quick and painless.

At the time of childbirth, **after the mother is admitted to the labour ward or when the labour pain starts,** the following treatment will ensure painless delivery within 20/30 minutes.

**Methods for Painless Childbirth :** Roll the pulley vigorously on the back of the two arms (from nails to elbow) for 15/20 minutes. The pulley is in the form of a grooved

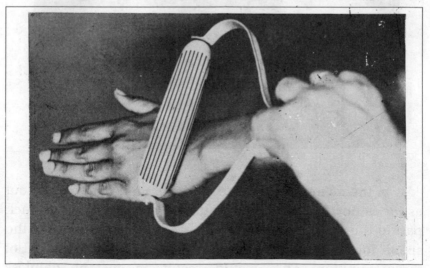

Fig. 72

wooden roller or plastic rollers. If such a pulley is not available, rolling can be done with grooved wooden rollers. Otherwise, the back of the two palms or the soles can be rubbed continuously from nails to wrists with two metal combs. Continue the rubbing for 5/8 minutes. There is no cause for worry even if the back of palms and soles become blood-red. If necessary, vaseline may be applied on the affected area after the delivery *(See fig. 72)*.

Afterwards ask the expectant mother to hold these combs between the tips of her fingers and the upper part of the palms joining the fingers as shown in the Fig. No. 73 and ask her to give a steady pressure on the comb with her fingers and thumbs for two minutes and leave it for 2 minutes and continue this. If other things are normal, the child will be born within 20 to 30 minutes and afterwards the mother will not feel exhausted.

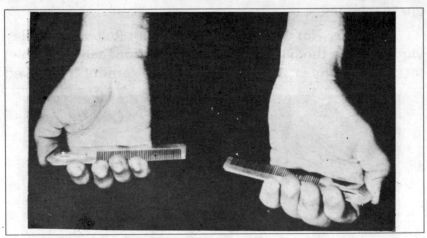

Fig. 73

In the meantime, ask the mother to take the tongue out as far as possible and give continuous pressure on the back part of the tongue (beyond the teeth) with the handle of the spoon for one minute. Repeat the same with an interval of three minutes. This would result in instant painless childbirth *(See fig. 74)*.

A *lady social worker of Bombay informs that the daughter of her relative took this type of treatment and within 25 minutes delivered a baby without pain.*

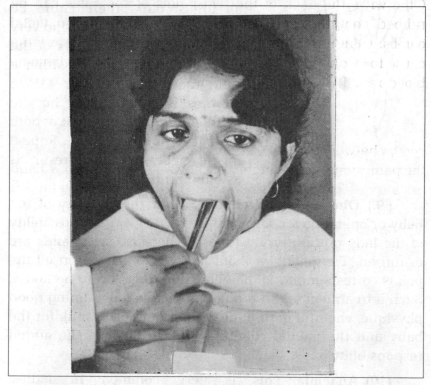

Fig. 74

( 7 ) **Difficult Labour :** Press hard on the inner side above the ankle as shown in figure 75 for 2 minutes and then pause and press again this way, till the child is born.

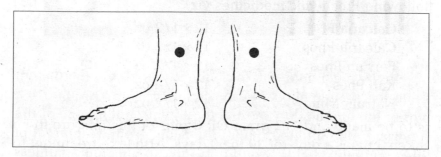

Fig. 75

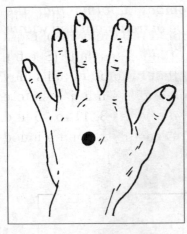

Fig. 76

**( 8 ) Pain in Breasts :** After the birth of the child, if owing to any reason it (the child) is not fed on breast milk, there could be accumulation of milk causing very severe pain in the breasts of the mother. For curing this within a short time, treatment for 4 to 5 minutes is to be given on the middle portion of the back of both the palms as shown here. Repeat this if necessary. The result is astounding (See fig. 76).

**( 9 ) Obesity after Delivery :** After the delivery of the baby or operation for sterilization, there is a great possibility of the lady putting on fat (obesity) because sex glands are disturbed. Treatment on Point Nos. 11 to 15 and on all the points corresponding to the endocrine glands is to be taken. Such a treatment taken regularly ensures maintaining good physique, cheerful nature, proper production of milk for the baby and the mental calmness needed to face the added responsibility.

**(10) Anaemia :** This is very common in ladies. Treatment on Point No. 37 together with supplementing the diet by green juice and health drink at least twice a day will show good results.

In acute cases, the mixture of powders/pills of the following Biochemic medicines viz :

| | |
|---|---|
| Calcaria Fl. | $12 \times 1/2$ oz |
| Calcaria Phos | $12 \times 1/2$ oz |
| Ferrum Phos | $12 \times 1/2$ oz |
| Kali Phos | $12 \times 1/2$ oz |
| Natrum Mur | $12 \times 1/2$ oz |

is to be made and 1/2 gram OR 3 pills of this mixture to be taken 3 times a day–for 30 to 60 days. Also take treatment to increase Haemoglobin as mentioned on page 244.

**(11) Falling of Hair :** This is a great problem especially with women. In such cases they should rub the nails of eight fingers against each other for 10 to 15 minutes daily (See fig. 77). For better results, it is advised that rubbing of nails may be done five minutes in the morning and five minutes before retiring. Moreover, give treatment on points 8, 11 to 15 and treatment to remove excess heat from the body as mentioned on page 262 (a) & (b) may also be taken. If there is a gynec problem, please cure it. Refer to pages 235/237.

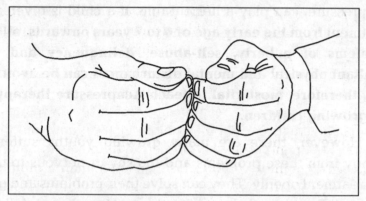

Fig. 77 : Picture showing rubbing of nails of eight fingers

**(12) Delaying Grey Hair :** As soon as the first grey hair is seen, start rubbing of the nails as mentioned above. The hair will remain black for a longer period.

**(13) Pimples :** These are due to scanty, irregular menses and excess of heat in the body. Treatment should be given on Point Nos. 11 to 15 and treatment for removing excess heat as mentioned on page 262 should be taken.

Regular use of this health science (Acupressure) will help the women to maintain good physique, achieve mental happiness, prolong their interest in sex, curtail their expenses on medicine and unnecessary beauty care, make their life happy and **make their home a Sweet Home.**

# CHAPTER 12

# MEN'S PROBLEMS

The problems of men usually result from an unbalanced development due to the disturbances in the sex glands. These are noticed at the time of puberty. Every child must therefore be given proper knowledge about sex, so that at the time of growth, that is from the age of 10 to 21, he can understand the changes occuring in his body and control them. Here, Acupressure, can play a helpful role. If a child is given this **treatment from the early age of 6 to 7 years onwards, all the problems of puberty, self-abuse, delinquency and the resultant physical and mental disturbances can be avoided. It is, therefore, most vital to teach Acupressure therapy to the growing children.**

However, there are many growing youths suffering silently from these problems and too shy or nervous to take the treatment openly. They can solve their problems and gain self-confidence simply by taking this treatment especially on Point Nos. 11 to 15 and all the points of endocrine glands. **Even in the case of those youths who are normal, this treatment will prevent them from going astray.** It should be remembered that semen is not meant for wasting.

After the age of 17/18, if semen is discharged in dreams once in a while, there is no need to worry. However, if it becomes regular, it requires proper treatment. Just as raw clay pots are put into a furnace and treated with heat; if semen is preserved properly till the age of 24 or more till marriage, sex problems after marriage could be avoided. Further, this properly cultured semen will be the basis of good, virile health. Also, it is the basis of spiritual development.

The same treatment is useful and effective in all the problems relating to less sexual desire, less satisfaction, etc. **In short, this treatment is useful wherever hormone treatment is necessary. (Point Nos. 11 to 15)**

**Less Desire/Less satisfaction/Early ejaculation :** The root cause of all these problems may be masturbation before marriage. The cause could also be excess heat in the body which causes thinning of semen. And this is discharged in sleep during erotic dreams and then through urine – called discharge of Albumin. To correct this problem do as under :

(a) Control sex as per fig. 80 and reduce frequency of intercourse.

(b) Remove excess heat as mentioned under 2 (a) and 2 (b) on page 262.

(c) Take treatment on all endocrine glands twice a day.

(d) Drink daily two glasses of gold/silver/copper/iron charged water reduced from four glasses of water for 60/120 days.

(e) Drink 2 to 3 cups of green juice adding in each cup 1 teaspoon of health drink and 1 table spoon of honey.

(f) Take "FIVE PHOS." 6 or 12, 3 – 3 pills in morning and evening.

(g) Treatment may be taken on the points shown in the figures No. 78 & 79.

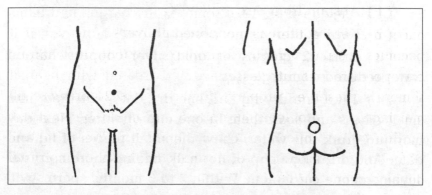

Fig. 78          Fig. 79

Moreover, after the age of 45–50, this treatment on Points 11 to 15 is useful in maintaining the heat of the body, controlling the prostate gland and thereby preventing hernia, old-age weakness and insomnia and overcoming all the problems of male climactory (known as menopause for men).

People following the spiritual path, if disturbed by erotic dreams and discharge, can successfully try this treatment on Point Nos. 11 to 15 and control shown below.

**Control :** Take a rubber ball of about $1\frac{1}{2}''$ to $2''$ diameter (like a tennis ball.) Place it under the seat between anus and testicles when loose clothes are worn. Sit on the ball for 5 to 10 minutes twice a day. This method can be tried by women also and is very effective in leucorrhoea *(See fig. 80).*

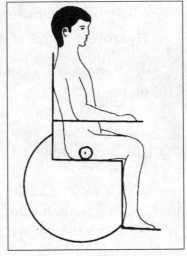

Fig. 80

**How to increase Spermatoza in semen :**

( 1 ) Abstain from Sex.

( 2 ) Keep control as mentioned above.

( 3 ) Drink 2 glasses of gold/silver/copper charged water reduced from 6 glasses.

( 4 ) Take one dry fig and one dry date; cut them into small pieces and soak them in one cup of water. Next day morning drink this water. chew the small pieces of fig and date. And drink one cup of hot milk adding therein crystal sugar and one cardamom. Within 2 to 6 months sperms will increase to normal level.

**Fertility :** In about 75 % of the cases, where the couple does not have a child, even after 3 to 15 years of marriage, it is found that the problem is with the husband. The above mentioned treatment is found useful and can be taken by both. This treatment surely increases the sperm count, corrects hormonal imbalance and increases the possibility of getting a child. In all such cases, it is advisable to take treatment to remove the excess heat from the body and also for V.D., Cancer of prostate or uterus (for females), H.I.V., if any. (shown under useful hints. Page 262–2 (a) & (b)).

**Hydrocele :** One of the root cause is weak digestive system and the other root cause is excessive sex. The valve allowing cerebro spinal fluid to enter into the testes and allowing this fluid to go back becomes weak. And so the fluid which enters testes does not go back properly is retained in the testes and the testes become bulging.

**Cure :** Do the treatment and exercises as mentioned for Hernia. Page No. 205. Also whenever you go to the toilet, squeeze the testes and wash them with cold water.

Also press on point Nos. 11 to 15.

You will be able to control this problem and prevent operation.

## CHAPTER 13

# HOW TO PREVENT OLD AGE AND MAINTAIN YOUTHFULNESS

**Problems of Ageing :** Death is certain. But everybody would like to maintain good health till the last breath.

The current of Life *(Chetana)* is discharged from the body from the right arm. The control point of this current is one inch circle on the front part of the right arm between the wrist and the elbow. By giving two minutes treatment i. e. intermittent pressure on this point, the excess discharge of *Chetana* is controlled. This will enable all to maintain youthfulness for a longer period and delay old age. This treatment is a MUST for all men and women after the age of 40.

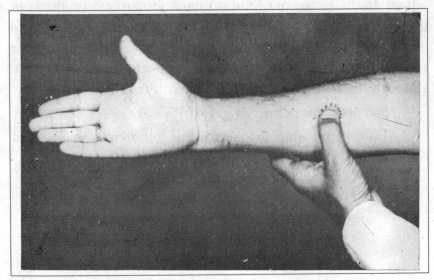

**Fig. 81**

It is interesting to note that **regular treatment on this point even by aged people will greatly benefit them and they will start feeling more energetic, younger and less tired.**

**Planning :** Now, that you have learnt how to prevent old age and remain youthful, it is almost necessary to have proper plans for the retirement. Activities of your choice must be increased, new hobbies common to both or complimentary to each other must be developed. Start taking interest in reading, writing and fine arts, music, painting, gardening, etc. Moreover move around a lot and see the world and meet people. You will feel a sense of oneness with them.

The most important is that, up till now, your activities were centred around you; start taking interest in others' welfare and find new avenues of great joy. Reduce your expectations and try to fulfill others expectations.

**Food :** It is observed by the medical world that after the age of 60 years, the heart and liver start functioning slower and slower. As such, rest after meals is most necessary. And a change in diet is a MUST. Try to reduce cooked food as much as possible. Increase the intake of green juices, fruit juices, green salads, fruits, yoghurt, etc. which are easily digestible and which will give you enough energy. Moreover, light exercise, Pranayam, walking/ swimming for 30/40 minutes are a MUST. Very soon you will be near Nature and every morning will bring you new joys and new meanings of life. And you will feel young, sing merrily like a bird and will feel confident, of living for 100 years.

# CHAPTER 14

# TREATMENT OF COMMON DISEASES

**The cycle of diseases :** You may kindly note that no disease or illness develops overnight. Most of the diseases and illnesses are caused by the breach of the laws of Nature, ignoring her signals, wrong habits of eating and drinking, bad habits of smoking and drinking, excess working of organs and the neglect of fundamental rules of hygiene. The illness starts in the body in the following manner :

( 1 ) There is less urination and so, more toxins accumulate in our body.

( 2 ) The fire in the stomach becomes weak. You get less appetite, so food is not digested properly resulting in constipation or loose motions.

( 3 ) Owing to the above two reasons, blood is not produced in adequate quantity and it gets impure.

( 4 ) When the blood is not oxygenated properly, carbon dioxide and toxins are not cleared from the organs and are not thrown out of our body.

( 5 ) Carbon dioxide and toxins collected around vital organs do not allow the current of life electricity to penetrate and recharge the organs. That is why malfunctioning or disease develops around that organ and it starts reflecting on thé palms or soles.

( 6 ) Accumulation of carbon dioxide and toxins lead to the slow functioning of the organs, reduction in vitality and increase in fatigue.

( 7 ) In short, our body gets weak and becomes prone to germs or diseases.

( 8 ) If a disease is prolonged, it affects the endocrine glands and the first endocrine gland to be disturbed is Thyroid / parathyroid gland. As these glands are interrelated, the damage to one gland leads to the malfuctioning of the other glands also. That is why in the case of prolonged illness, you find pain on the points related to more than one endocrine glands.

Nature wants our body to throw out the toxins, foreign matters or disease-causing germs. Acupressure helps our body in that work. When you press the points, a powerful current is sent to the corresponding part of our body thereby trying to clear the carbon dioxide and toxins collected around the organ and make the organ function effectively. These toxins go to the kidneys and so after giving treatment on other points, it is necessary to give treatment on Point No. 26 pertaining to the kidneys.

**Language of our body :** Before starting the treatment, we must also know the language of our body, that is, the meaning of the signals it gives.

( 1 ) We are well aware of the signals for thirst, hunger, urination and motion.

( 2 ) The body also gives us a signal in the form of belching when the stomach is full. We get the first call, it is followed by a second call and a third call.

( 3 ) Ache or pain in any particular part shows congestion of carbon dioxide, water, air, etc.

( 4 ) The running nose and sneezing mean that the body is trying to throw out excess water.

( 5 ) Coughing indicates that
    ( a ) the body is feeling cold and that
    ( b ) it is trying to clear congestion in the throat and
       the chest.

( 6 ) Itching shows that a greater flow of blood is required around that part.

( 7 ) Fever indicates the battle in our body i.e. white blood cells are having a fight with the germs of a disease.

( 8 ) Twisting of the body indicates that it is tired and requires rest and oxygen.

( 9 ) Loss of appetite indicates that there is congestion and constipation and that the stomach and other digestive organs are busy in removing the congestion or the constipation or the body is busy in fighting the disease. In such a case only lukewarm water and fruit juices or buttermilk should be taken instead of further taxing the stomach with food.

(10) Pain or murmur in the heart indicates that the heart requires total rest. The best way is to remain in bed for 24 to 72 hours and take treatment on all the points including Nos. 1 to 5 and 36.

We should understand these signals of our body and try to help our body to get rid of the disease and never try to stop these signals suddenly by any drugs e.g. sudden stoppage of fever has many times resulted in some other disease, even in paralysis.

**How to recharge the inner battery :** In order to get faster relief and break the vicious cycle of diseases as mentioned above, it is advisable to do the following to recharge the inner battery.

( 1 ) Perform Pranayam.

( 2 ) Drink lukewarm water, preferably copper/silver/ gold charged and health drink.

( 3 ) Skip a meal or two, reduce the solid food intake and take fruits, vegetables juices and buttermilk, thereby allowing rest to the digestive system.

( 4 ) The battery of our body is recharged during sleep. So it is most important to have good sleep whenever you feel tired or when there is pain on more than 2 to 3 points on the palms or soles.

The above four things help to recharge our unchange- able battery. **This battery is capable of curing almost all the diseases.** And that is why it is most important to recharge this inner battery.

**Before treating any disease, the root cause must be found and removed :**

( 1 ) First, check up whether the Solar Plexus is in order or not. If it is not in order, please get it in order (Refer to pages 73 to 76).

( 2 ) Secondly, see that the nervous system passing through the spinal cord is in order. This can be checked as under :

Lie down on the stomach. Keep the arms straight on sides. In the lower lumbar, you will observe two shallow round depressions on both sides of the spine as shown in the fig. 82. If this is the case, the problem in the body is not due to the nervous system connected with the spinal cord. If you find such depression only on the right side, then the problem is on the left side and connected with the spinal cord. Similarly, if the depression is on the left side, there is some problem with the right side, connected with the spinal cord. The sciatic nerve, about a quarter inch thick which starts from

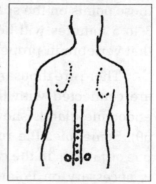

Fig. 82

the brain goes all the way down to the lower lumbar and then is divided into two. It then, reaches the heels and the toes. The whole nervous system is connected with this sciatic nerve which gets the protection of the spinal vertebrae. Now if, for any reason, there is pressure on any part of this sciatic nerve, the nervous system connected with that part is impaired and results in some problem or the other *(See fig. 20 & 22)*.

So, if you find that any of these two shallow depressions are not seen, check up the spinal cord. Run two fingers from the first cord of the vertebra and go on till the last. If you observe that some vertebra is lower, that is the root cause of the trouble. e.g. if Point No. 4 vertebrae is found lower, it can cause stammering. If Point Nos. 6 to 9 are not in order, it can

cause pain in chest which sometimes is mistaken for heart attack.
To put the vertebra in the proper
position, rub it upwards by
pressing from both the sides of
the spinal cord as shown in the
figure 83.

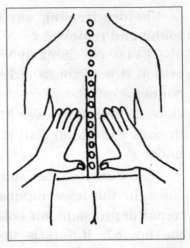

Fig. 83

Secondly, give treatment on
the point of the sciatic nerve
shown in figs. 42 (a) and (b) of the
feet. Thirdly, karate chops around
those points on the spinal cord for
3 to 5 minutes will help to bring
that vertebra in proper position.

There are thousands of names of diseases but all of them
are connected with the malfunctioning of the organs and
endocrine glands shown in figs. 39 and 40 (see pages 66 to
69). Sometimes the root cause may be found in more than
one organ e.g. in the case of bronchitis and asthma treatment
is necessary on Points 1 to 7, 34 and 30 because the root
causes of these diseases are cold and weakness of the lungs.
With a little experience, you will be able to find out the points
where it pains. And so, after recharging all the organs by
pressing each palm or sole for five minutes daily, treatment
is to be given only on those points where it pains.

**Health Powder / Drink :** In 300 grams of amla powder,
add 100 grams of dried ginger powder. Mix them. Take one
teaspoonful of this powder along with water in the morning
and evening.

Otherwise, in 4 glasses of water add 2 tea spoonfuls of
the above powder of amla and dried ginger (use fresh amla
and ginger if available) and boil it and reduce it to 3 glasses.
Filter the water and drink it during the day. If desired, honey
can be added to it. This is good for growing children.

Amla is a concentrated vitamin 'C'. It has 16 times more vitamin 'C' than the lemon has. Such a drink will give protection to the body against cold and increase digestive power. It is of astringent (तुरा) taste and not sour.

People in the West take apple cider which is also beneficial. The health drink is beneficial to all, especially to the convalescing people, old people, expectant mothers and growing children.

**Green Juice :** Our body requires energy to function properly and to throw out toxins and diseases. This juice has all types of salts and minerals required by the body and this juice is easily digestible. Such green juice was given to patients of blood cancer, in which cases weight goes on reducing regularly. Even though green juice has very less calories, these patients gained weight from 2 to 4 kgs. per month just by drinking 3 to 4 cups of green juice per day. It is pure energy. (thicker the leaf, more is energy in it.) From experience, it has been found out that leaves of any non-poisonous plant / tree could be used.

To prepare such green juice, one can take :

Leaves of tandaljo/spinach, methi (fenugreek), cellery, lettuce, cabbage, green coriander, pudina (mint), tulsi (holy basil), even cucumber, radish, simla capsicum, wheat grass and sprouted cereals, etc. In short, use leaves of any nonpoisonous plant/tree and vegetables from which juice can be extracted. While preparing such green juice, add one amla when available in the season or add dry amla powder/dry ginger powder also. (amla has 16 times more Vitamin C than an equal size of lemon.)

In case, such green leaves are not available, dry leaves can be used. In that case, soak such dry leaves in water for two hours. Then throw away the water and extract juice.

PLEASE CLEAN THESE GREEN LEAVES THOROUGHLY BEFORE USING THEM.

Such green juice is PURE ENERGY. Those who desire to lose weight, should take 6 to 8 cups of such juice in a day +some fruits only. They can lose 7 to 10 kgs. of weight per month without any side effects. And those who desire to increase weight / height, should also drink 3 to 4 cups of such green juice but add one table spoon of honey to each cup.

It is possible that till toxins are cleared from bowels / intestines, one may get loose motions when they drink such green juice. Afterwards, such loose motions will automatically stop.

This green juice is a MUST for sick people, growing children, expectant mothers and old people. It has no side effects and can be taken by patients having kidney problems.

Such green juice will make you EVERGREEN.

**Green Paste :** While preparing such green juice paste / pulp will be available. Do not throw it. Add little turmeric powder and cream of milk to it and apply it on the face or any part having skin problem/even on white spots as a MASK. Take blue light on it for 6 to 8 minutes. After 15 minutes, wash with water, and see the wonderful result just in 15 days.

**Copper/Silver/Gold and Iron charged water :** It has been found that the following minerals are useful for treating diseases connected with the organs as shown below :

**( 1 ) Copper :** Useful for all diseases and problems connected with the nervous system e.g. high B.P., arthritis, polio, tension and leprosy.

**( 2 ) Silver :** Useful for diseases of the organs connected with digestive system and the urinary system.

**( 3 ) Gold :** Useful for disorders of the breathing system, lungs, heart, brain and is a general tonic.

**( 4 ) Iron :** Proper quantity of iron in blood is utmost necessary because they carry oxygen and supply it all over the body and thus increases stamina.

### The charged water can be prepared as shown below :

Take a pot of Pyrex glass, if possible; otherwise take a copper vessel, if readily availabe. In that case copper is not to be included while boiling. Otherwise stainless steel vessel or even earthen pot can be used. Do not use Aluminium or brass vessel.

( 1 ) **Copper charged water :** Put 60 grammes of pure copper plate / ingots / wire or 6 to 8 copper coins in 4 glasses of water and boil it.

( 2 ) **Silver charged water :** Put 30 to 60 grammes of silver-pure bullion or pure coins (.999 purity) in 4 glasses of water and boil it. Do not use silver ornaments.

( 3 ) **Gold charged water :** 15 to 30 grammes of gold pure bullion gold coin or ornaments (chain or bangles not enameled of 22 carat gold in 4 glasses of water and boil it).

( 4 ) **Iron charged water : (In case of deficiency of iron in blood, anaemia or during pregnancy**) Put 60 grammes of unrusted piece of iron (nails, etc.) in 4 glasses of water and boil it.

**All these metals can be put together in water,** in the proportion of gold 15 to 20 grams / silver 30 grams / copper 60 grams / iron 60 grams. It should be borne in mind that all metals put in the water are thoroughly cleaned and **do not contain any dust or rust.**

Boil away 25% of water i.e. retain 3 out of 4 glasses of water after boiling. Filter this water, keep it in a thermos if possible and drink it lukewarm / hot during the day. Drinking of 1 glass of such water the first thing in the morning is very beneficial. When this water is reduced by 50 %, it becomes medicine – best antibiotic and is a MUST in treatment of all serious diseases. In acute cases, this water may be boiled down to 1 glass or even half a glass. When you drink such concentrated water (i.e. when more than 60% water is boiled away e.g. 3 glasses of charged water reduced from 8 glasses) avoid sour things like lemon, sour buttermilk, etc.

The charged water is found useful for good health. But it is a must for the treatment of any problems connected with the improper flow of the current of bio-electricity i.e. high B.P., polio, rheumatism, arthritis, paralysis, chronic diseases including cancer, etc. The use of concentrated gold charged water has given wonderful results in the case of mental retardation, muscular distrophy, T.B., heart attack, etc., and is a good brain tonic too.

**Quantity :** The above quantity is for all above 12 years. For children over 2 years 50 % of the quantity is to be given. For children below 2 years give only $\frac{1}{4}$ quantity.

**Treatment for Common cold, cough, flu, fever, tonsils, etc. :**

The above mentioned common diseases are the biggest enemy of mankind. They are responsible for the highest number of working hours lost. Though they are not deadly, they make you most miserable. The common cold causes headache, coughing, sinusitis, tonsilitis, fever, bronchitis and when neglected may result even in deadly pneumonia. We must properly understand our body and ascertain the root cause of this common cold.

As mentioned earlier, our body consists of about 72% of water. Heat and cold have the same effect on the water inside our body as on the water outside. Our body also has an airconditioner as well as a heater. In summer or in winter, it maintains the temperature of 98.6° F (36.9°C). The water in our body gets heated during the day due to activity and due to outside temperature, while during the night, it cools down, creating moisture in the lungs or head. In Nature, it is thrown out in the form of dew. In the case of our body, it is thrown out by sneezing or watering of the nose in the morning. Therefore, sneezing in the morning is considered to be a sign of good health.

During the year the body tries to throw out excess water twice through sneezing and running of the nose, which is known as common cold. The phenomenon lasts for 3 to 5 days each time. One need not worry about such cold or try to stop it. It is jokingly remarked that in common colds if you take medicine, you will be all right within 6 days but if you do not take medicine you will be all right within 4 days.

Further, the water in the blood and the body is controlled by heat. The heat of the body depends upon one's digestive power. So whenever the digestive system weakens the internal temperature goes down. This reduces the evaporation of water and gathering of excess water in the body. In turn this excess water reduces the heat, resulting in the congestion in the lungs, chest and throat. Whenever this water gets congested in the head, it causes headache. This cycle leads to tonsilitis, sinus trouble, bronchitis and fever. The excess of water is aggravated by cold drinks, heavy foods, sour things like curd, buttermilk, lemon and by exposing the body to cold winds or coldness through air-conditioning. All these add to the prolongation and aggravation of the disease.

**Effect of the moon on the body :** The moon is the satellite of the earth, and being very near to the earth, it has great effect on the water on the earth. The obvious proof of this is that the time of high and low tides changes daily alongwith the moon day.

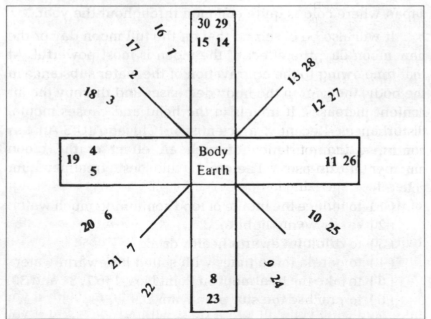

Fig. 84 : Rotation of the Moon round the Earth

From the figure 84 about rotation of the moon around the earth, you will observe that on the 4th, 5th, 8th, 11th, 14th, and 15th, 19th, 23rd, 26th and 29/30th of moon- days, the earth and our body come directly against the moon. At that time the water level in the sea and in our body rises. And so, on these moon days, in the Indian religions, particularly, in Jainism, people are advised –

( 1 ) to observe complete fast, (not to drink even water, if possible) or

( 2 ) to eat only once, or

( 3 ) to eat only twice, or

( 4 ) at least to avoid eating green vegetables (as they contain about 90% water) and thus control the water in the body, thereby reducing the chances of cold.

People suffering from chronic colds or sinus trouble or having allergy to cold should try to carry out as many of the above restrictions as possible. Moreover, these restrictions can be observed on a national scale in countries like U.K. and Japan where cold is quite common throughout the year.

It will also be observed that on the full moon day or the new moon day, the effect of the moon is most powerful. At that time owing to the aggravation of the water substance in the body, the heat in the body decreases and thereby the air content increases. It travels to the head and causes mental disturbances. Recently, a scientist in Chicago (U.S.A.) has confirmed the existence of such an effect of the moon on mental diseases. Therefore, the best treatment for cold is –

( 1 ) to reduce the intake of food containing much water.

( 2 ) to eat warm, light food.

( 3 ) to drink lukewarm health drink.

( 4 ) to gargle three times with salted lukewarm water.

( 5 ) to take the treatment on Point Nos. 1 to 7, 34 and 30.

( 6 ) to practise the sun pranayam.

**Cold due to Heat :** The other reason for headache and cold is sluggish liver. As a result of less biles, the food is not turned into alkali and so the acidity in the stomach and intestine which is called 'Pitta' (पित्त) increases. That leads to the warming of air in the stomach. This heated air occupies the empty spaces in the head and the face. Now during the day, whenever this heated air is cooled, due to the cold wind, the running of fan over the head or sitting in an air conditioned place, it gathers moisture and becomes water. This cooled water contracts the nerves leading to headache and sinus trouble. When the accumulated cold starts coming down, it irritates the throat and the nose and leads to tonsils and causes sneezing and running of water through the nose. In such a cold, the chest is clear. Now, in such cases of cold, any pain reliever upsets the stomach and in the long run leads to ulcer and hyper-acidity. It is observed that this type of cold is aggravated in summer and autumn. At such a time, when pressed, there is a pain on Point No. 28 of the Adrenal gland.

The best way to remove this excess of heat from the system is to take Harde powder (हरित की चूर्ण) (powder of Terminalia, Chebula Retz). In 2 to 3 grams of this powder add 1 gram of sugar. Take this the first thing in the morning with lukewarm water. This may cause one or two loose motions. This treatment is to be continued for a week, and afterwards only once or twice a week. If such powder is not available, drink one glass of water or fruit juice or one cup of green juice the first thing in the morning after cleaning the mouth.

Secondly, all points connected with cold are to be pressed i.e. Nos. 1 to 7, 30 and 34.

Thirdly, the points of the Adrenal gland, liver, gall bladder, stomach and Solar Plexus i.e. Point Nos. 28, 23, 22, 27 and 29 are to be pressed.

Fourthly, in the case of an old complaint, it is useful to take the following medicine for 4 weeks. It helps the digestive system.

Nux Vomica 200-4 pills twice in a day but once a week

Nux Vomica 12 or 30- 3 to 4 pills }  (Homeopathic
    twice daily                   }   medicine)

It is claimed by The Indian Ayurvedic Science that Harde powder is not habit-forming and can be safely given to small children duly mixed with honey. This can solve many a problem connected with constipation. Moreover, it is claimed that if Harde powder is taken regularly for 45 to 60 days the first thing in the morning and lukewarm water is drunk throughout the day, it helps a lot in reducing the fat in the body. During such a course, light food is to be taken only twice a day, after having at least two loose motions.

Fifthly, take out excess heat from the body by any of the methods shown at the end of this book, under 'useful hints.' page 262 – 2 (a), 8 (b).

## COMMON COMPLAINTS

Acupressure treatment for some of the common ailments is given below. If necessary, the treatment may be supplemented by Ayurvedic or Homeopathic/Bio-chemic medicines and other treatment also mentioned herein.

**( 1 ) Cold and Cough :** This is a very common complaint occuring either due to a change in the climate or owing to indigestion, overfeeding and consuming of raw sugar. Treat on all points twice daily plus Point No.1 to 7, 30 and 34, and in the case of children, Point No. 38 also. Please give the child only lukewarm water to drink and give the treatment for constipation.

**( 2 ) Blocked Nose :** In case of cold and sinus, many times the nose gets blocked. Take treatment for 2 to 3 minutes on the point of forehead and on the point on both the sides of the nose for immediate relief. (See the figure)

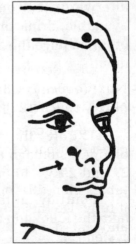

Fig. 85

If possible put a drop of lukewarm ghee (boiled butter) in each nostril at the time of retirement.

**( 3 ) Bronchitis Pneumonia-Flu and Hay Fever :** When there is not enough heat in the stomach and so food is not digested properly, it turns up into phlegm which rises up in the wind pipe goes into brocili of lungs. In order to remove the same, body brings coughing and in case of too much congestion, one gets fever and it is declared as bronchitis. If not treated in time, it can develop into Pneumonia and Hay fever. For cure, do as under :

( 1 ) Stop cold food-like milk, curd, cold stored foods, fruit juices, canned juices and icecream and anything with sour taste.

( 2 ) Add a little salt and a pinch of turmeric powder in half a glass of lukewarm water and drink it the first thing in the morning. Do again the same way in the afternoon and evening. This may cause vomiting, which is helpful to remove congestion.

( 3 ) When hungry, eat only light hot meals.

( 4 ) Drink 2 glasses of charged water reduced from 4 glasses.

( 5 ) Keep Solar Plexus in order to remove constipation.

( 6 ) Take 2 to 4 cups of green juices adding there in each cup 1-teaspoon of Health drink (atleast ginger powder)+1 tablespoon of honey.

( 7 ) Remove worms, if any, and take Nux Vomica 200 3/4 pills twice in a day but only once a week. Nux Vomica 12 3 pills in the morning and evening.

( 8 ) In case of heavy congestion, take Red Light on the chest and back for 2 to 3 minutes.

( 9 ) Put half ground bishop's seeds (अजवाईन) in a tablespoon-fill it only half. Then put lemon juice on it to cover it fully. Do this after sunrise. Keep this for at least two hours and eat it but definitely before sunset. Within ten days, Eosinophilia will come under control.

**All types of fevers :** For any type of fever except typhoid, take the following treatment :

Put clothes pins and rubber bands on Points No. 1 to 7 and 34 as shown in fig. 86 and keep them for 5 to 10 minutes. Then remove them for 15 minutes. Then continue in this manner till the fever comes down. In most cases fever comes down within 15 to 30 minutes.

In case of malarial fever, also give treatment on Point No. 37 and also take 1 teaspoon of "Sudarshan choorna" (Ayurvedic bitter medicine) in the morning and evening.

During any types of fever, drink lukewarm water half a glass every half an hour. If possible drink charged water.

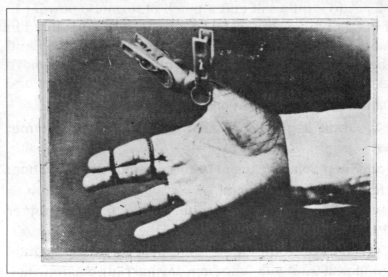

Fig. 86

**( 3 ) Bronchitis, Pneumonia, Flu and Fever :** When there is acute congestion in the chest or throat, Nature causes fever, even bronchitis and pneumonia. Take the same treatment as in (1) above. In case the fever is due to malaria, Point No. 37 should be pressed. And take only lukewarm water boiled with black pepper and salt.

**( 4 ) Whooping Cough :** Press Point Nos. 1 to 7, 30, 34 and 38. Give boiled, lukewarm water added to ginger, turmeric powder and salt. Give pressure on the first knot of the middle finger of both the hands. (See the figure) Correct Solar Plexus.

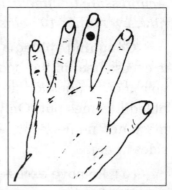

**Fig. 87**

**( 5 ) Sinusitis :** Apply pressure on tips of fingers and toes, and also take the treatment mentioned in (1) above. Also take the treatment to remove excess heat– as per page 262–2 (a), 2 (b).

*Mr. 'G' had chronic sinusitis trouble. Even an operation couldn't cure him. During the night, he had to keep his mouth open in order to breathe. He started this treatment and on the fourth night, he slept with his mouth closed. And within a fortnight his complaint was totally gone.*

**( 6 ) Tonsilitis :** Press Point Nos. 1 to 7 and 34. Please see that the mouth and throat are cleaned, Gargling with lukewarm water with a little salt aded to it three times a day is also advised. Tonsilitis shows that the heat of stomach is reduced and so lukewarm water and light food are to be taken. **In cases of swollen tonsils, apply turmeric powder on the tonsils, then gargle with lukewarm water with a little salt added to it and then apply Glycerine Tanic Acid inside the throat and gargle with salted lukewarm water.** There is no necessity to get the tonsils removed. Get rid of constipation. Whenever possible, drink lukewarm water and take Acupressure treatment.

*Mr. 'B' reports that he had been suffering from tonsilitis, cold and cough since he was quite young. He did not get the tonsils removed by operation but he had to take injections when he got fever every 30 to 40 days. Since he started this*

*Acupressure treatment, his complaints have disappeared and now, even after 10 years, he enjoys good health.*

**Coughing – phlegm coming out :** It happens when there is excess heat in the body and digestion also becomes poor, you feel congestion in throat and with every coughing phlegm comes out. Only one treatment is not enough – you must not neglect but attack such problems from all the sides ... e.g.

(a) Remove excess heat as per 2 (a) & (b) on page 262.

(b) Remove worms, if any.

(c) Take a course of Nux Vomica for 45 days.

(d) In the morning, at noon and in the evening, take the treatment mentioned above for Tonsilitis. That will remove a lot of phlegm from the throat.

(e) Keep in the mouth a small piece gum + a piece of crystal sugar; that soothens the throat and prevents coughing. Do so 4 to 5 times.

(f) After every meal, chew a little of bishop's seeds (अजवाईन) adding to it little quantity of sugar.

**( 7 ) Loose Motion, Diarrhoea, Dysentery :** This is a clear indication of overeating and indigestion. Reduce diet, drink plenty of lukewarm water adding some ginger, lemon and barley to it. Acupressure treatment is to be given on the feet and palms on Point Nos. 19, 20, 23, 25, 27 and 38 and in the middle of the chin for constipation. Correct Solar plexus.

From the age of 7 months to 18 months, loose motions may be due to teething, if not cured by the above mentioned treatment, the child may be given more of calcium. preferably 2 to 3 pills of Calcaria Phos 12×3 times a day. For patients exposed to heat, loose motions can be due to excessive heat. In such a case, over and above the points mentioned above, treatment may be given on all the tips of fingers and toes and Point Nos. 1 to 4.

**( 8 ) Diarrhoea and Cholera :** Over and above the treatment mentioned above for severe problems, for a mild attack take treatment for 3 – 4 minutes twice a day on the point below the knee-cap as shown in the figure.

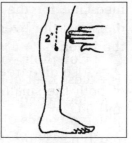

Fig. 88

**( 9 ) Intestinal Worms :** When pressed on the point on the outer side in the middle of the smallest toe/last finger, if pain is observed, it is an indication of worms. This is a common problem with children. Wherever children complain of pain around stomach, and loss of appetite and their growth has stopped, then first of all try and find out about worms. In case of worms, the children even get ear infection and in such cases point of Lymph gland no. 16 will be found paining.

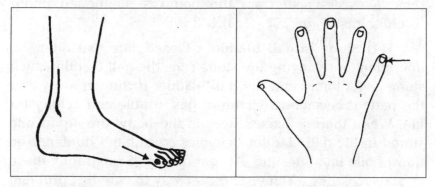

Fig. 89                                         Fig. 90

In such cases, the worms have to be removed. Give patients Cina 200 (A Homeopathic medicine).

For children

| Under 6 | Under 10 | Over 10 |
|---------|----------|---------|
| 4 pills | 6 pills  | 8 pills |

Once a day for 4 day. Then, stop medicine for 4 days. After 4 days repeat the medicine as mentioned above.

On the 13th day, give some powerful laxative and afterwards give Cina 12 – 3 pills for 30 days. If allopathic medicine is taken for worms then supplement it with medicine for the liver – because such medicine for worms damages the liver. Also give treatment on Point No. 23 of the Liver.

Also give treatment for 3 minutes twice a day on points of both the small fingers or small toes, as shown in fig. 89 and 90.

In case of ear infection remove worms and give treatment for the same as shown on page 192. The same treatment for worms, has been found useful in an Athelete's foot i. e. fungal infection of skin.

**(10) Jaundice and Liver troubles :** For jaundice and other liver troubles, press Point Nos. 19, 20, 22, 23, 25, 27, 28 and 38. Stop taking oily and heavy food. Remove cream from milk before drinking it. Eat gram, chew sugarcane or drink its juice, eat dates and have buttermilk and curd. Also remove excess heat from the body as mentioned under 'useful hints'. Page 262 – 2 (a) & 2 (b).

**(11) Stone in gall bladder :** Please note that after the operation for removing the stone from the gall bladder, such stone is not found and the gall bladder is thrown away and the patient becomes a victim of gas trouble and acidity for life. When there is excess heat in the body, the liquid bile stored in the gall bladder becomes crystal and hinders free flow of bile into intestine. At that time, in Sonography these crystals look like a stone. The best way to cure this problem is to remove excess heat as per 2 (a) – (b) of 'useful hints' on page 262 and to take a cup of green juice adding there to one teaspoon of health powder +1 tablespoon of honey 3 to 4 times a day; +2 glasses of fresh fruit juice + treatment as mentioned under (10). Also give Blue light on liver / gall bladder for 5 to 6 minutes twice a day.

Even in case of severe damage to liver in advanced stage of jaundice, when liver is feared to have burst, this treatment has been found to be very useful and it prevents surgery and lifelong misery.

**(12) Hyper–Acidity :** Sometimes you wake up with an unpleasant taste in the mouth, heaviness in the head, a burning sensation in the stomach and a feeling of nausea and vomitting. These signs indicate hypertension / liverishness. In such cases, take treatment on the point on the outer side of the leg, one inch above the ankle, as shown in the figure for 3 to 5 minutes. Plus treatment to remove excess heat as mentioned on page 262–2 (a) & 2 (b). Also eat 2/3 pieces of clove or blackpepper after meals.

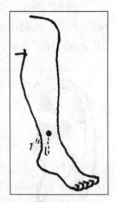

Fig. 91

Further do the following for long term relief :

( 1 ) Remove excess heat as mentioned under 2 (a) and (b) on page 262.

( 2 ) Give pressure treatment on Point No. 22, 23 & 28.

( 3 ) Half–an hour before meals, eat a mixture of half teaspoon of cumin seed powder जीरा + half teaspoon of sugar.

( 4 ) After meals, chew 2 to 3 cloves or black pepper.

( 5 ) Avoid constipation.

( 6 ) Drink 2 to 3 cups of green juice.

( 7 ) When you feel uneasy due to too much acidity, burning sensation, do as under :

(i) Chew 2 to 3 pieces of black pepper with a pinch of sugar.

(ii) Drink 3 to 4 table spoonfuls of cooled milk, every 15/20 minutes. If soda is available, add 3 to 4 tablespoonfuls of it to this cooled milk and drink it every 15/25 minutes till burning sensation stops.

( 8 ) In case of heaviness/pressure on chest due to gas, correct Solar Plexus and press on inside border of Point No. 8.

Try to find out root cause which could be even damage to brain. Then take the treatment as mentioned on page 249.

**(13) Epilepsy/Fits :** Treat all the points and all the points of endocrine glands, viz., Points 1 to 4, 8, 14, 15, 25, 28 and 38. Try to find out root cause.

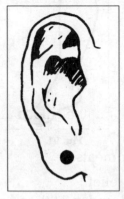

**Fig. 92**

**(14) Convulsion :** In the case of children having convulsions, press gently on both the ear lobes as shown in fig. 92. Within half a minute, the child will become normal. This is an instant treatment. Try to find out the root cause. It may be due to damage to Pituitary/Pineal gland or even to the brain. In such cases, treatment on all the endocrine glands plus 1 glass of gold/silver/copper charged water reduced from 4 glasses is necessary. In serious cases, take treatment for brain's problem (page 249).

**(15) Fainting :** Repeated attacks of fainting can be due to serious problems as mentioned above. Try to find out the root cause and give the treatment accordingly. For instant temporary relief, press on point as per fig. 93 on the small fingers of both the hands and on point No. 36.

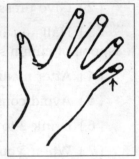

**Fig. 93**

**(16) Teething :** Press on all points especially on Point No. 8. Also give the baby 4 pills 3 times a day from the following mixture :

$$\left.\begin{array}{l}\text{Calc. Phos } - 12 \times \\ \text{Calc. Flour} - 12 \times \\ \text{Fer. Phos } \quad - 12 \times \\ \text{Kali. Phos } - 12 \times\end{array}\right\} \ \frac{1}{2} \ \text{oz each}$$

Mix them.

Start giving these pills when the baby is 4 to 6 months, that will enable easy teething.

**(17) Crying of Children :** In case a child cries due to fear, irritation or not being able to sleep, give treatment on all tips of the fingers and toes and back of both the palms or soles.

**(18) Overgrowth of the body :** Treat all the points daily + Point Nos. 3, 4, 8 & 38.

**Undergrowth of the body :**

( 1 ) Treat all the points twice daily + all the points of endocrine glands.

( 2 ) Drink two glasses of charged water daily reduced from 4 glasses.

( 3 ) Drink two to three cups of green juice adding to each cup 1 teaspoonful of health powder & 1 tablespoonful of honey.

While preparing the green juice, add 25 % sprouted cereals like Mung (मुंग).

( 4 ) Check as regards worms and remove them, if necessary.

( 5 ) Stop any bad habit if any, cure discharge of ova and semen. i. e. cure problem of white discharge and masturbation.

( 6 ) Do regular exercises. Expose yourself to plenty of sunlight. Do Pranayam as much as possible (page 112 – 113).

**(19) How to increase Height and Weight :** Even if the parents are not tall or even below normal; the height of the children can be increased up to the age of 20 years. However, such efforts should be made at the earliest. Take the following treatment :

( 1 ) Take treatment on Points Nos. 3 – 8, 11 to 15 – 25 – 28 & 38 for children below 15.

( 2 ) Take 1 glass of gold/silver/copper charged water reduced from 2 glasses (up to the age of 7 – 8) and then 2 glasses reduced from 4 glasses of water.

( 3 ) Take about 75/100 grams of sprouted pulses (मुंग – चना) daily. It should be chewed thoroughly. Jaggery/ sesame (तील) can be mixed with them.

( 4 ) Drink 1 to 2 cups of green juice daily adding therein carrots and ginger plus honey.

( 5 ) Do exercises as shown in fig. 23 for correcting spinal cord, at least 8 to 10 times.

( 6 ) Also do exercise on single-bar, jogging, swimming & yogic exercises.

( 7 ) And refrain from abuse of sex – i. e. masturbation. Girls must see that they have regular menses.

( 8 ) With this treatment, even **weight** will increase and become normal.

**(20) Wetting the bed :** Press all points plus Point Nos. 11 to 15, 18 and 26. Also press the first and second knots of the last finger of both the hands. See the figure 94.

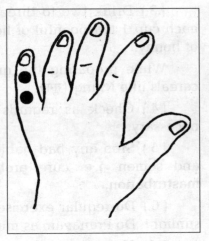

*An American Doctor's nephew and niece had this problem. After they unsuccessfully tried all the forms of treatment, they began giving Acupressure treatment to them. Within a week, these children stopped wetting their beds.*

**Fig. 94**

**(21) Urinary troubles (like less urination or stone) :** Press all points and Point Nos. 11 to 15, 18 and 26. Also press the first and second knots of the last finger of both the hands (see fig. 94). Also apply cold pack on the abdomen.

Drink at least 6 to 8 glasses of water to promote free and regular flow of blood. This will help the kidneys to function properly and to throw out poisons from the body and you will have clear urine.

For all the problems connected with urinary troubles, urinary track, including stones, the combination of the following Ayurvedic drugs has been found very useful :

( 1 ) 100 grams of powder of seeds of Eugenia Jambolana (Jamun ke Beej).

( 2 ) 100 grams of powder of Bombax mala baricum-root (Shimla ke Mool).

( 3 ) 10 grams of powder of Asphalt (Shilajeet) – (These are available at Ayurvedic Shops).

8 to 10 grams to be taken every day the first thing in the morning.

**(22) Failure of Kidneys :** When toxins in the blood cannot be removed through kidney, they gather there and hinder the function of kidneys. More and more toxins gather. The level of Kreatine in the blood increases. This condition is known as **Pyletis** and patient is asked to go for dialysis; after a few months, the patient is advised to go for transplantation of one kidney. Surprisingly, nobody bothers to find out the root cause of excess toxins. Do not panic. Do the following :

( 1 ) Press all points for 5/6 minutes on each palm + press Point Nos. 3, 4, 8, 11 to 15 + 16, 25, 26 & 28 – 3 times daily for 1 – 1 minute each.

( 2 ) Drink 2 glasses of silver charged water reduced from 8 glasses of water. This helps in reducing excess heat and activates the kidney.

( 3 ) Drink one cup of black tea, the first thing in the morning. In case of nausea keep 2 cloves or little sugar in the mouth. After 15 minutes, regular breakfast can be taken.

**How to prepare Black Tea :** Put 1 teaspoon of leaf tea (any tea will do) in one cup of water. Boil till it becomes half cup. Filter it and add half a cup of ordinary water (not from refrigerator). Drink it hot for 12 to 15 days.

**How to find out whether Kidney has started functioning properly :** On the first day before you start drinking Black Tea, take your first urine in a glass. It will be observed to be hazy and having bad odour. On the 12th day or 15th day, take the first urine and check it. When the urine is found to be clear and without bad odour, it denotes that kidneys have started functioning normally.

**How to prevent failure of Kidneys :** Even healthy persons can make a habit of drinking such black tea for 12 days every year – preferably in cold climate. And forget worrying about problem of kidney.

**Stone in Kidney :** When Thyroid/parathyroid glands do not function properly, the calcium in our food is not digested properly and it is calcified and when it cannot be cleared in urine, it gathers in kidney and forms a stone. In such a case, the above mentioned treatment will be found very useful. Stone will get crushed and be removed in 10/15 days. Continue the treatment on Point No. 8 and other endocrine glands. When there is no pain when pressed on Point No. 8 it denotes that thyroid/parathyroid glands have started functioning normally and so new stones will not be formed. It may be noted that in case it is Acetate stone (hardly in case of 10 %) it may not be removed with the above treatment. But such cases are rare.

*Several patients living on dialysis or those who were advised transplantation of kidney, have successfully tried the above method.*

**Root cause : It may be noted that in all cases of kidney problems, always try to find out the root causes and treatment to remove such root causes MUST be taken alongwith above mentioned treatment.** In about 90 % of the cases examined by me, I have observed that in case of males, the root cause was venereal diseases, cancer of prostate or HIV developing into AIDS. And in case of females, it is the cancer of uterus, HIV in advanced stage.

*Case Study : One lady of about 35 years of age, came to our Free Centre at Arya Samaj, Santacruz(W). She was advised to have transplantation of kidney. Luckily, her mother's kidney was found to be suitable/matching and so the operation was to be performed only after ten days. On examination, I found that the root cause was cancer in uterus. She was asked to postpone the operation for just 45/60 days.*

*She started taking the treatment for cancer of uterus + above mentioned treatment for kidney. She started passing normal urine just in 10 days. After 45 days, she went to the same doctors who had advised her to go for transplantation of kidney. The doctors were surprised with the healthy condition of the patient and declared that she was in good health. Her kidneys were of normal size and functioning properly and as such there was no necessity for the operation for the transplantation of kidney.*

Similarly, I have helped avoid over 200 such operations for the transplantation of kidney. Thousands of patients have been happy to stop dialysis. And in the same way, thousands of patients have been able to have the stone removed from their kidneys with the above mentioned treatment.

**(22) Skin Diseases :** These are not diseases but symptoms showing lack of Vitamin C and indigestion due to sluggish liver, resulting in impure blood. Certain foods mixed and eaten together create poisonous substances in the body and if this poison is not removed from the body by the kidney, it comes out in the form of eruption on the skin, known as skin disease. It is, therefore, advisable not to eat cereals, fish, onions, garlic, citrus fruits and antibiotics along with unwarmed milk, curd and butter-milk. The first urine in the morning can be applied on the affected parts to ensure early cure. Treatment on all the points together with more Vitamin C (amla, lemon, fruit juice, raw vegetables) groundnuts and til (seasame) in diet will soon cure the disease and also remove the problem of dry skin. Also take health drink (see page 168) Also take treatment to remove excess of heat as mentioned on page No. 262-2 (a) & (b). Check up Point No. 37, if it hurts immediately start treatment for cancer of the blood.

**(23) Boils :** Press the Lymph gland Point No. 16 on the middle of the wrist and also take the treatment on Point No. 26. Proper daily treatment will ensure that there are no boils and if there are any, they will soon dry up.

**(24) Anaemia :** Press all the points and Point No. 37, 3 times daily. In cases of chronic complaint, take medicine for Anaemia as advised in chapter 11. Also drink iron charged water and green juice. In case of serious problem also follow instructions given on page 244 to increase Haemoglobin.

**(25) Allergy :** Press Point No. 21 and take 3 to 4 Calcaria Phos 12x globules or tablets twice a day. Also take Kali Phos 12 or 30, 3 – 3 pills in the morning and evening. Follow this course of taking Cal. Phos & Kali Phos. for 45 days only.

**(26) Eyes :** For anything wrong with the eyes like pain, watering, reddishness, etc. give treatment on Point No. 35 and put a pack of cold milk or extract of kothmir (coriander leaves) on the eyes. Eat plenty of raw carrots or drink carrot juice. If regular treatment is given on these points after the age of 45, it will prevent cataract. Even during early stages of cataract, this treatment is very beneficial.

**This treatment can prevent "BLINDNESS" due to cataract. Moreover, even in case of Trachoma of eyes, operations have been averted with this treatment.**

**Serious Problems :** The optic nerve is governed by the pituitary gland. For any serious problems of eyes, check the Point No. 3 and points of optic nerve on the back of palms. (see fig. 41 (a) & (b)). If found to be tender, paining, give the treatment on these points as well as on Point No. 3 & 35. Also drink 1 glass of gold/silver/copper charged water reduced from 4 glasses of water. Also drink at least 2 cups of green juice.

**How to do away with spects/glasses :** It has been observed that up to minus number 3 to 4 (for seeing); with the help of following treatment, the eyesight becomes normal and one can stop wearing spects/glasses :

( 1 ) Press the Point Nos. 3, 22, 23 and 35 on both the palms 3 times a day for 2/2 minutes each. Give pressure

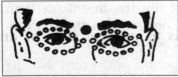

treatment around the eyes as shown in fig. 95 for 2 to 3 minutes on each eye 3 times a day. Pressure is to be given on the bones around and not on eye ball.

Fig. 95

( 2 ) Drink at least 2 to 3 cups of green juice which should include carrots and sprouted pulses like chinese green peas (मुंग) and health drink i. e. amla powder+ginger powder.

( 3 ) Do Pran Mudra as per page 114.

( 4 ) Reading must be done in a right sitting posture under proper light.

( 5 ) In order to prevent damage to the eyes, children should be taught from the beginning to read in a proper upright posture and view the T.V. from a reasonable distance. They should be taught how to blink the eyes regularly.

( 6 ) The mother should stop the use of hydrogenated oil/vegetable ghee/margarine at least 3 months prior to conceiving till the child is breastfed. If possible, there should be a total ban on the use of hydrogenated oil/margarine in the house. Such use creates excess of H+ in the brain which in turn damages the eyesight of the children, born and to be born.

( 7 ) Also blink each eye for 2/3 minutes in an eye glass filled with rose water or cooled self urine of morning or cold water.

( 8 ) Wherever possible take the sunrays directly in the eyes for 5 to 6 minutes within 60 minutes after sunrise or 45 minutes before sunset. If that is not possible, take blue light on the closed eyes.

Within 3 to 5 months, the eyesight will improve and become normal. Then, take proper care of eyes throughout the life.

For all the problems of eyes drink atleast one cup of green juice adding thereto 1 teaspoonful of health drink powder.

**Eye Drops :** The best thing is to put the eyes in an eye-glass filled with pure water and blink them for 2 to 3 minutes each or sprinkle fresh water on the eyes.          **OR**

To 8 oz. of rosewater add 1 grain of alum and put these drops in the eyes regularly.

**Eye Ointment :** Slightly rub black pepper on a clean stone surface with few drops of water. Apply this thin paste in the eyes. Even though there is a little burning, it clears up the eyes and increases the power of the eyes. Or apply ghee prepared from cow's milk in the eyes before going to bed.

**Cataract :** This can be prevented with the above mentioned treatment. For more details, read author's book "Health in Your Hands: Volume 2."

Also in the morning while in bed, apply your own saliva in the eyes. Drink daily one cup of green juice/carrot juice.

**(27) Ears :** For any pain or pus or noises in the ears, points 31 and 1 to 3, 34 and 38 should be pressed. For pus give treatment on lymph gland (Point No. 16).

**Ear drops :** Urine is the best form of ear drops. Otherwise, take 60 ml or 50 gm of edible oil. Put 1 peel of garlic in it. After the oil is warmed up, filter it and keep it in a small bottle. Use it as ear drops when necessary.

**(28) Deafness :** This is not hereditary in most cases. If mother has sinusitis, cold, mumps, etc., during pregnancy, it affects the ears of the child in the womb and so sometimes the child is born deaf.

However this deafness can be cured :

( 1 ) Just check up as regards worms and clear them. The method is explained earlier on page 181.

( 2 ) In case of pus in the ears, give treatment on Point No. 16 of lymph glands; also put 2 drops of hydrogen peroxide 2/3 times a day & clean the ears. Then put 2 drops of ear drops as mentioned above.

( 3 ) Give treatment on Point Nos. 1 to 6, 31 and 30 – 34 three times a day for 2 minutes each.

Do not worry if cold increases. In such cases give the patient lukewarm water to drink.

( 4 ) Give 1 glass of gold/silver/copper charged water reduced from 2 glasses.

( 5 ) First give yellow light on each ear for 2 minutes. Then give blue light on the ears for 5+5 minutes in the morning and in the evening.

( 6 ) On the spot of wisdom tooth, pressure may be given by cotton/rubber studded wooden stick or by chewing there soft clean rubber/eraser.

The results are amazing. Continue the treatment for further 30 days even after recovery.

*Mr. D aged 60 had lost his hearing power for 5 years. He was given treatment on Point No. 31 of ears. To his astonishment, within a month, he was able to hear.*

*A baby aged 7 was reported to be deaf since birth. She was given this treatment. Within 60 days improvement was noticed and normalcy was restored within 120 days.*

**(29) Dumbness :** Dumbness is mostly due to deafness. So treat such patient for deafness and press the tips of all the fingers and toes. This treatment can also be given when the patient is not able to speak clearly or stammers. In such cases, please give treatment on vertebra No. 4 of the spinal cord (Page 168, fig. 83).

**(30) Hiccough :** Press hard on the back of the first knot of the middle finger as shown in fig. 87 for whooping cough, or bring the tongue outside the mouth as far as possible and hold it in the same position for 1 to 2 minutes. Check the Solar Plexus and correct it if necessary.

**(31) Sunstroke, Heatstroke, Fainting, Bleeding through the Nose :** Take the treatment on tips of fingers and toes and press hard on the point below the nose and above the upper lip as shown in the figure.

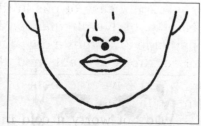

**Fig. 96**

Practise Moon Pranayam. For longterm cure, give the treatment as per 2 (a) & (b) as mentioned on page 262.

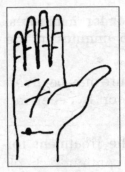

Fig. 97

**(32) Palpitation :** Press the point as shown in the figure at the corner of the wrist and palm of both the hands, for 2 weeks.

**(33) Water Worms :** In case there is a hole (mouth) apply wet *Multani Matti* (available with all Ayurvedic druggists) around the mouth. Within a short time, the worm will start coming out. Roll it on a pencil and very slowly pull out the worm. Please be careful to see that the worm does not break. The worm can be 6 to 8 inches in length. In case there is no mouth or hole, eat the following for 4 to 8 days. Take a bitter-gourd, clean it and roast it on fire. Afterwards eat it like boiled corn. If necessary, salt and lemon can be applied. Eat for 4 to 6 days, there will be an opening.

**(34) Hysteria :** Give pressure on the inner first joint of the thumb as shown in the fig. 98. Check about cancer in uterus and, if necessary, take the treatment as mentioned on page 237.

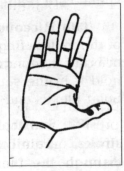

Fig. 98

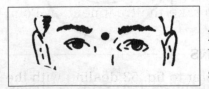

Fig. 99

**(35) Dizziness and Severe Pain in Sinus :** Press the point between the two eye-brows as shown in fig. 99.

**(36) Loss of Voice or Sick Voice :** Press inside the thumb with the other hand at the point shown in the figure. If it continues, take the treatment as mentioned for Tonsilitis and remove excess heat.

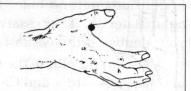

**Fig. 100**

In spite of this treatment, if the problem continues, check up Point No. 16 and if it is pains, do the treatment for cancer of the throat as mentioned on pages 239–240.

**(37) Corn :** Massage the affected part with ice for 2-3 minutes. Afterwards, rub turpentine oil on it and bandage it. In the morning, this corn will come out. Afterwards, continue rubbing turpentine daily for 2 to 3 days. Rolling of feet on a wooden roller has been found to prevent further formation of corns. Give the treatment on Point No. 8.

Also take 4 pills in the morning and 4 pills in the evening of the mixture of Calc. Phos 12 × and Calc. Flour 12 × for 3 months.

**(38) Fatigue :** Under fatigue conditions, do not eat anything. Drink lukewarm gold/silver/copper charged water or health drink. If this is not available, drink one glass of lukewarm water at intervals of half an hour.

Also give this treatment : Take a small comb, preferably of metal and keep it in the right hand as shown in fig. 73 and press it with the thumb on the side of the comb and with fingers on the comb. Press it hard on the upper part of the palm joining the fingers. After half a minute, do the same with the comb in the left hand and repeat the same treatment after one hour, if needed. Also take the treatment on Point No. 32 of energy.

## PAINS

**(39) Toothache :** Please refer to fig. 53 dealing with the aching tooth. Give the treatment on that fingertip In the case of severe pain, press this tip of the finger continuously for more than 2 to 3 minutes. Remove the pressure when the finger starts getting blue. Then treatment can be continued again, later on, if necessary. It could be due to cavity. So see your dentist at the earliest.

Also take 2 pills in the morning and 2 pills in the evening of Calc. Phos – 12 × and Calc. Flour – 12 × each for 3 months.

**(40) Bodyache :** Pain in any part of the body without an external cause clearly shows that the battery of the body has become weak, and that the flow of air is locked up there. So, one must do the needful as mentioned earlier to help the battery get recharged. The pain is due to the fact that carbon dioxide and cold have accumulated in that part. So, the best cure is to take copper/silver/gold charged lukewarm water at least 3 to 4 glasses in 24 hours and to give Acupressure treatment on all the points. In such cases, 'sudarshan' powder has been found to be very effective. Take half a teaspoonful of this powder, add half a teaspoonful of turmeric powder mixed with half a cup of lukewarm water and after drinking it, drink some more lukewarm water.

If the bodyache continues, press on Point No. 37 of spleen. If it pains when pressed, it could be serious. Read author's book "Defeat The Dragon" chapter on HIV/AIDS. Do not neglect. Please note that it is curable.

**(41) Headache :** Most of the headaches are due to cold, change of season, etc., resulting in congestion in the head and can be cured by treating Point Nos. 1 to 7 and 34. Also practise sun Pranayam.

Sometimes headache is also caused by heat where the liver is affected or by overworking of pancreas resulting in migraine. In such a case, the treatment on Point Nos. 23, 25 and 26 will give good results. Also practise moon Pranayam. Also remove excess heat as per 2 (a) & (b) as mentioned on page 262.

Sometimes headache is due to some trouble connected with the eyes or tension in the neck. In such a case the Point Nos. 35 or 7 should be pressed.

In cases of very severe pain, continuous pressure can be given on finger 1 and 2 and thumb with the help of clips or rubber bands, which must be removed before the fingers become blue *(see fig. 52)*.

If it continues in spite of all the above treatment, it could be serious. See fig. 115 and press on point 3″ above the earlobes of both the ears and if it pains it could be some problem in the brain. Treatment for the same is given in the next chapter.

**Migraine :** If there is severe headache but only on one side, it could be due to overworking of Pancreas gland. Do the following :

( 1 ) For temporary relief, eat 100 grams of Jilebi (जलेबी) (an Indian sweet) and drink sweet hot milk as the first thing in the morning for only three days. If jilebi is not available, eat some sweets (100 grams).

( 2 ) Press on all the endocrine glands, each for 1 to 2 minutes, three times a day.

( 3 ) Drink 2 glasses of charged water reduced from 4 glasses.

**(42) Back Pain :** Please note that Point No. 9 is on the back of the palm. It starts below the thumb and the first finger and goes down till the middle of wrists, called Point No. 16–lower lumbago. The whole line is Point No. 9 and pressure is to be applied on that, for treatment. see fig. 41 (a) & (b) also see (45) below :

*What Dr 'P' reports, sounds almost like a miracle : "I got rid of the problem of stiff back in the morning with regular practise of Acupressure. When one of my friends came to see me, I thought of trying the same on him as he was stooping and regularly complained of backache. I took his hand in my hand and went on pressing on Point No. 9 for about four to five minutes. When my wife entered the hall, he got up to say "Hallo" and, to the surprise of all, he was standing straight and there was a great relief from backache. My friend thought I had performed some miracle. Now my friend is an ardent follower of Acupressure therapy."*

**(43) Pain in the Legs :** Roll your feet for 2 to 3 minutes on the grooved wooden roller as shown in fig. 69.

**(44) Sciatic nerve :** When this nerve is pinched awkwardly and constantly, there is pain in hips, thighs and legs. Treatment is to be given on the points related to sciatic nerve shown on the back of the palms and the lower portions of the legs as shown in fig. 41 (a) & (b) and 42 (a) & (b). It has been observed that faster relief is obtained by giving treatment on the points of the sciatic nerve in the legs for about 5-6 minutes.

A lady dentist had severe pain in the right leg and thigh for a long time. She had taken many X-rays and other treatments, without success. She consulted an Acupressurist. He found the points of sciatic nerve to be tender and suggested treatment accordingly. Within 10/12 days, she was cured.

**(45) Knee Pain :** Treatment is to be given for 2/3 minutes thrice a day on the points shown in fig. 101.

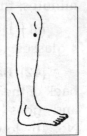

Fig. 101

Also check the sciatic nerve points. If it pains, give treatment on points of sciatic nerve as shown in fig. 42 (a) & 42 (b).

In case of continuous severe pain, apply the following paste for only 6 to 7 minutes in the evening.

Take an equal quantity of turmeric powder (हलदी) + Bishops seed (अजवाईन) + Garlic (लसुन) and grind them to make a paste. Apply it around the knees and wash it after 6 to 7 minutes and if burning sensation is felt, massage coconut oil on the knees.

**(46) Problem of Slip Disc – Severe Pain in the back, spondylitis, thighs, both the legs, kneepain etc :**

In the first chapter, importance of sciatic nerve, the cable cord of our central nervous system is explained. Now, it is possible due to several reasons, like falling down, severe jerk, faulty way of sitting, etc., any of the vertebrae might have pinched into the spinal cord thereby causing a serious problem. In such cases, the patient has to wear a collar or waist band, lie down for a long time in a sandbox, keep hanging heavy weight on the legs. Swelling in that point in spinal cord is taken as slip-disc and many a time the operations are advised in such cases. The severe pain in the back spreads to the legs through the sciatic nerve and the patient finds difficulty in walking. In all such cases, the following treatment may be tried before going for an operation.

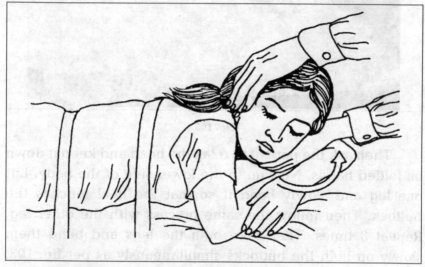

**Fig. 102**

Take a cushioned bed $1\frac{1}{2}$ to 2 feet wide and 6 to 7 feet long and 18 to 30 inches in height. Ask the patient to lie down on stomach and keep a soft small pillow (14″ × 14″) under the chest. Then, 3 strong straps are to be tightened – one as much high as possible between vertebrae No. 5 and 9. The second one is to be tightened in the middle of the buttoks and third one is to be tightened on the middle of spinal cord. These straps are to be tightened as much as possible so that the body does not move but not so tight that the patient finds difficulty in breathing (see fig. 102).

Then take the head of the patient in both the hands and rotate it slowly but steadily and with as much pressure as possible in a round, circle, upper, sideways, down the other side and rotate it for 3 to 4 times without giving jerks as per fig. 103.

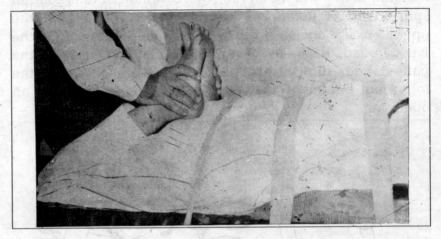

**Fig. 103**

Then ask the patient to relax the head and keep it down on folded hands. Now go to the lower side of the body. Lift one leg and slowly bend it so that the heel touches the buttock. Then follow the same process with the other leg. Repeat 3 times. Then take both the legs and bend them slowly on both the buttocks simultaneously as per fig. 103. In the first sitting do not give more pressure. The patient may find pain, may cry out in agony for half a minute. But afterwards, there will be great relief as the sciatic nerve gets freed.

If necessary, repeat this treatment after one to two days. With only 2 to 5 sittings, in most of the cases, the patient will get cured. If not, the patient can consult an osteopath or an orthopaedic surgeon. If the patient has already undergone an operation of the spinal cord or the knee within one year this treatment should not be taken.

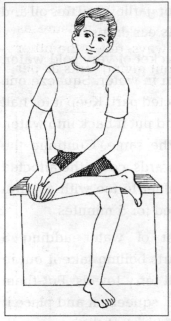

**Fig. 104**

Sit on a chair. Keep left foot firmly on the ground. Then keep right leg on the knee of left leg as shown in fig 104. Then with two hands try to press down the right knee three to four times. Repeat same way with the other leg.

**(47) Muscular Pain and Fibrosis :**

( a ) Give treatment on the tips of corresponding fingers.

( b ) Massage the affected part lightly with :

( 1 ) Regal medicated oil and embrocation available in Hongkong, Singapore and in big Indian cities like Mumbai, Chennai and Kolkata, which can be prepared at home by mixing the following :

| | | | |
|---|---|---|---|
| Menthol crystals | 25 % | Methyl Salisylate | 15 % |
| Camphor powder | 10 % | Eucalyptus oil | 10 % |
| Oil Lavenarspike | 7 % | White oil | 33 % |
| (If not available use | | (or kerosene) | |
| Enca Pyptusoil) | | | |

This is good for massage on the affected parts of paralysis, polio and severe muscular pain.

**OR**

( 2 ) Mixture of Edible oil (80 %) and
Eucalyptus oil (20 %)

**OR**

( 3 ) Edible oil + ginger powder or garlic. (Boil this oil and keep it in a bottle. It is also useful as ear drops.)

**( c ) Cold Pack :** Take half a bucket of very cold water. Take 2 small terry towels, soak them in water. Squeeze one of the towels and place it on the affected part. Keep it for half a minute. It will dry up. Remove it and put it back into water. Take the other towel and repeat the same. Continue the treatment for 5 to 10 minutes. Afterwards, cover the affected part and the whole body from shoulder to toe with a warm woollen blanket. Keep it thus covered for 5 minutes.

**(d) Hot Pack :** Boil 1 bucket of water adding 3 tablespoons of salt to it. When it starts boiling take it out in a wider tub or utensil. Take 2 small terry towels. Put them into the water. Take out one of them, squeeze it and place it on the affected part for 1 minute and repeat the same with the other towel. Continue the treatment for 5 to 10 miutes. Afterwards, dry up the affected part and cover it; do not expose it, for 10 minutes.

**( e ) Blue Light :** Before 10 a.m. or after 4 p.m. hold blue glass against the sun and 18 inches (45 cm) away from the affected part. This is a blue light.

**OR**

Take a 60 watt blue bulb. If it is not available, wrap 4–fold blue gelatine paper around a regular 60 watt bulb. Light the bulb and keep it 18–20 inches (45–50 cm) away from the affected part for 10 to 15 minutes at a time.

**( f ) Red Light :** Instead of blue glass or blue gelatine paper, take red glass or red gelatine paper and do similarly as mentioned above. But red light is to be given on affected parts for only two minutes. Useful in paralysis/Polio.

**( g )** Similarly, yellow light is useful in deafness.

**(48) Chest Pain :** There are several reasons for chest pain, which is often mistaken for a heart attack. In the case of a heart attack, you will find pain on pressing Point No. 36. If there is no pain on that point, there is no cause for worry. Give treatment on the middle of the back of the left arm as shown in figure 105 for 3-5 minutes.

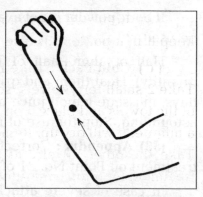

Fig. 105

**(49) Stomach Pain and Gas Trouble :** First check up Solar Plexus and put it in order if it is not. Check up about worms as mentioned under (9) of this chapter and remove them. Give pressure on Point Nos. 19, 22, 23 and 27.

**(50) Pain Reliever :** For all types of pain, the following treatment gives instant temporary relief :

Take a little of common salt. Heat it on a pan till it becomes red, brown or dark grey in colour. Keep it in a bottle. Put about 1 to 2 grains of such salt on the tongue every 5 to 10 minutes till the pain subsides. Do not go on repeating more than 4 times during a day. If this salt is taken at night, it causes sleep. However, be careful not to take this salt in excess or to form the habit of taking it.

**(51) Swelling :** First check Point No. 26 of kidney. If there is pain, take treatment as mentioned in this chapter for Pyelitis / kidney troubles. However, if there is no pain there, it means that the swelling is local. In that case, take some rice. Grind it into powder. Add little turmeric powder. Boil this powder in half a cup of milk till it turns into a paste. Apply this paste as much hot as bearable on the affected part and keep the bandage on the same. Repeat it for 3 to 4 days. It will be cured. Also check point 36 of heart.

**(52) Ring Worm :** After bath, massage the dried affected part with Dettol or antiseptic lotion. Then, massage the part with dry boric powder for 3 to 5 minutes.

If boric powder is not available the following powder can be used.

Half of alum + half of borax (टंकणखार) (Both in equal quantity). Heat them and grind them into powder. After 3/4 days, massage lemon juice on the affected part. Results are astounding. Stop the use of nylon and plastic panties.

**(53) Appendix :** Correct the Solar Plexus. Give treatment on Point No. 21 of the Appendix.

In case of severe attack, there will be severe pain in stomach so that the patient tosses from side to side. At that time, press little hard in the middle of calves. That will be painful but it will soon cure the problem.

Also give continuous pressure on Point No. 21 for more than 3 minutes.

Later on, give treatment on Point No. 21, 19 and 27 for complete cure. Take 2 to 3 cups of green juices. 1 to 2 glasses of fruit juice and green salads, etc. Avoid foods of fine flour, fried food, etc.

**(54) Vericose Veins :** (see fig. 69) Sit on a chair. Keep the roller on the floor and roll the soles on it for 5 to 10 minutes in the afternoon and at night before going to bed.

For those persons, in whose family there is a history of such problem and those who have to stand for long periods, this treatment should be taken to prevent the problem of vericose veins and of pain in the legs.

Moreover (a) treatment on Point Nos. 3 – 4 – 8 – 11 to 15 – 25 – 28 and 36, (b) Drinking of 2 glasses of gold/silver/copper/iron charged water reduced from 4 glasses of water, (c) and doing Sarvangasan (fig. 122) twice a day for 2 to 5 minutes is found to be very beneficial. This problem could be due to a weakened heart. Check Point No. 36 of heart and if it hurts, take treatment for heart as mentioned under (8) in the next chapter. Do not neglect.

**(55) Hernia :** When the stools become sticky or hard, extra force is required to throw out the stools. At that time, Apan Vayu is kicked back and irritates the intestines. When such a thing becomes regular feature, the intestine muscles near the thigh becomes weak and bulging like balloon comes out on either side near the thigh. This bulging comes out while exerting stools or when the Solar Plexus moves down or also when the patient is standing or walking for more than 10 minutes or more.

**Cure :** ( 1 ) The best way is to improve the digestion and see that the stools is not sticky and easily extracted and is such that it floats on the water. If necessary make changes in the diet-stop eating heavy foods which are not easily digestable. Eat more vegetables and drink green juice. If necessary add fibre like "SAT ISABGOOL" and take mild laxative before going to bed.

( 2 ) Remove worms, if any + treatment on points 11 to 15 + Correct Solar Plexus, which may have shifted downwards.

( 3 ) Take a treatment of Nux Vomica for 45 days as mentioned in the book on page 126.

( 4 ) Take a mixture of ginger powder half a spoon + Sudarshan powder half a spoon twice a day for 45 days.

( 5 ) Do the following exercises preferably on empty stomach or atleast 3 hours after meals.

**( a ) Pull ups :** Lie down on back-keep spongy pillow under the head. Lift the head as much as possible and maintain that position for 10-12 seconds and repeat for 15 to 20 times to start and slowly reach doing this pull ups for 75 to 100 times. See the figure below.

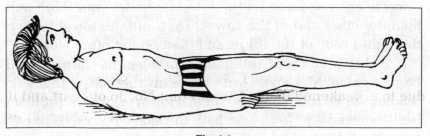

Fig. (a)

( **b** ) Lie down without pillow. Then with both the legs do cycling – when you bring down the legs, bring them as slowly as possible and when the legs are six inches from the ground, try to maintain that position as much as possible. Do such cycling for atleast 30 to 40 times. See fig. below.

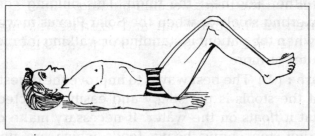

Fig. (b)

( **c** ) Keep both legs touching the buttocks. Then raise the body as shown in the figure. Then with both hands, rub vigourously the corners of thigh towards the abdomen for the one minute to two minutes. See fig. below.

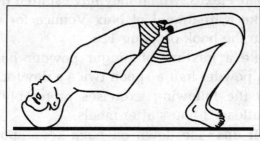

Fig. (c)

( **d** ) While passing stools, press hard on the part where there is ballooning.

( **e** ) After bath, while standing, keep one end of the towel in one hand and let the towel go under your thigh and hold the other end of the towel. Then rub the towel first on the right inside of the thigh and then on the other side.

If this is followed religiously, problem of Hernia could be prevented. Moreover, with these instructions, if followed religiously, Hernia can be cured. However, if this problem has advanced and found on both the sides, it is advisable to consult the Doctor.

**(56) Hydrocele :** One of the root cause is weak digestive system and the other root cause is excessive sex. The valve allowing Cerebro spinal fluid to enter into the testes and allowing the fluid to go back becomes weak. And so the fluid which enters testes does not go back properly – is retained in the testes and the testes become bulging.

**Cure :** Do the treatment and exercises as mentioned above for Hernia. Also correct Solar Plexus. Also whenever you go to the toilet, sqeeze the testes and wash them with cold water.

Also give treatment on point nos. 11 to 15 and then all other endocrine glands.

Thus you will be able to control this problem and avert operation.

**(57) Emergency :** In case the patient finds it difficult to breathe, or has become unconscious or similar type of problem like stroke, brain haemorrhage, etc. has arisen; do not panic. Do the following :

( 1 ) Make the patient lie down on the floor.

( 2 ) Start pressing Point No. 36 of Heart and do so for two minutes like pumping and repeat after five minutes.

( 3 ) Press Point Nos. 1 to 5 on both the thumbs. Take three to four minutes to do so.

( 4 ) Press each earlobe for 1 minute.

Any type of attack will subside within 5 minutes. Then give one glass of hot water to drink (preferably charged water).

Give the patient 1 glass of fresh fruit juice (of any fruit available) or in case the fruit juice is not available, give him 100 grams of jaggery (गुड़) to eat. That will give him/her instant relief. During that day, no food is to be given – give the patient only liquids, charged water (from 4/6 glasses reduced to 2 glasses) + fruit juices + green juice. If possible give the patient enema with coffee powder. Next day, try to find out the root cause and give the treatment for the same.

---

# CHAPTER 15

# TREATMENT OF SERIOUS DISEASES

Besides the common diseases, discussed in chapter 14, there are some serious and sometimes contagious diseases which require special care. **The following treatment will be common for all of them :**

( 1 ) Give boiled water, preferably lukewarm+two to three cups of green juice adding health drink and copper/silver/gold charged water, 2 glasses reduced from 4.

( 2 ) Treat all the points including the tips of all the fingers and toes twice daily.

( 3 ) Give treatment on all the points of the endocrine glands twice a day for 1–1 minute each.

**Diet : This plays an important role in the cure of all serious diseases.** Follow the chart :

**6 a.m. to 7 a.m. :** Correct the Solar plexus. To remove excess heat, do as per 2 (a) & (b) as per page 262.

Then after 20–30 minutes, drink 1 cup of black tea as mentioned on page 187.

**7 a.m. to 8 a.m. :** Drink one cup of green juice adding 1 teaspoon of health powder+one tablespoon of honey.

**9 a.m. to 10 a.m. :** Fruits/Fruit juice.

**11 a.m. to 12 a.m. :** Green juice as mentioned above.

**1 p.m. to 2 p.m. :** Green salad as much as possible. You should add sprouted mung 75 to 100 gms. you may also add ground nuts+little jaggery and a pinch of black salt.

**4 p.m. to 5 p.m. :** Green juice ... 1 cup of curd/yoghurt (after 10–15 days when very hungry) adding a pinch of rocksalt in case of *Vat/Kapha Prakruti* or 1 teaspoon sugar in case of *Pitt Prakruti*.

**6 p.m. to 8 p.m. :** Fruits/Fruit juices.

During the interval, drink charged water and complete its quota. If desired drink more water, preferably hot to lukewarm.

**After 8 p.m. :** Nothing except water, if desired.

**Breathing exercises :** During the add as much as breathing exercise including Kapal Bhati and Bhastrika.

Over and above, further treatment should be given separately for different diseases as given below :

## TREATMENT

**( 1 ) Small Pox and Chicken Pox :** Press Point Nos. 22, 23, 28 and 38. Protect the patient from heat. Practise moon Pranayam.

**( 2 ) Measles :** Press Point Nos. 28, 30, 34 and 38. Take care against cold. Practise sun Pranayam. After 7 days, practise moon Pranayam and also take the treatment to remove excess heat from the body.

**( 3 ) Mumps :** Press all the points daily, including the tips of all the fingers and toes. Keep the throat clean by gargling. Practise sun Pranayam.

**( 4 ) Diptheria :** Press Point Nos. 6, 7, 16, 30, 34, 36 and 38. See that the mouth, especially tongue, is cleaned 3 times a day. Gargle with lukewarm water with a little salt added to it. Give the patient treatment for tonsilitis as mentioned in chapter 14. Practise sun Pranayam.

**( 5 ) Typhoid :** Press Point Nos. 19, 22, 23, 26 and 27 on the soles and palms. **Take proper care in diet, green and fruit juices and butter milk only – and take complete rest. Gold/silver charged water 4 glasses reduced from 16 glasses is beneficial and so is a MUST.** Practise moon Pranayam. Correct Solar Plexus and check it regularly.

( 6 ) T. B. : One gets this disease because of (a) long stay in damp air (b) absence of sunshine and (c) mal-nutrition. Hence, to cure this disease all these causes should be removed. Practise the following :

( 1 ) One must develop the habit of going to parks and places where one can get fresh air. There the patient should do sun Pranayam for 25 – 30 minutes as mentioned on page 111 and 116.

( 2 ) Wherever possible the patient must sit in sunlight for 30 to 60 minutes. But he should take care that he does not get cold draft of wind.

( 3 ) The patient must drink at least 3 to 4 cups of green juice, adding to each cup 1 teaspoonful of health drink + 1 tablespoonful of honey (if honey is not available, add jaggery).

( 4 ) (a) Take daily 2 glasses of fresh fruit juice.

(b) Moreover, twice a day ask the patient to lay down on back and open his mouth wide open. Pour one tablespoonful of honey directly in the throat in such a way that honey does not touch the tongue.

( 5 ) Ask the patient to drink 4 glasses of gold/silver/copper/iron charged water reduced from 16 glasses of water.

( 6 ) **Acupressure Treatment :** If the patient gets, cold, give the treatment for tonsils, continue all other treatments.

( 7 ) Give light of INDIGO colour on lungs and upper back for 5 to 6 minutes in morning and evening.

Just within 20 – 30 days, you will observe miracle. Even after, recovery, continue Pranayam, sunbath and green juice for life. Another root cause of this disease is smoking, working in unhygienic conditions. See fig. 113 and do accordingly to stop. Stop the habit of chewing or smoking tobacco. Stop masturbation and sex.

( 8 ) Also do Ling Mudra and Pran Mudra as per page 114 – 115 and sun Pranayan as per page 116.

**( 7 ) Gastro-enteritis/Dehydration :** Give only lukewarm water adding ginger, lemon, barley and honey as frequently as possible. Press Point Nos. 19, 22, 23, 26, 27 and 38 on the soles and palms. Correct Solar Plexus. Check for worms and remove them, if required.

**( 8 ) Heart Attack :** Heart is a muscular structure and supposed to work throughout one's life time. **When you have pain in the chest, please check Point No. 36 by pressing it. If there is no pain, it means that the cause for this chest pain is not in the heart. In that case :**

( 1 ) Check the Solar Plexus. If it is not in order, there could be gas trouble. Correct it.

( 2 ) It can be muscular pain starting from vertebrae 6 to 8. In such a case, give treatment for 3 to 5 minutes on the point of middle of the back hand as shown in the fig. 105. Later on, rub eucalyptus oil or pain balm on the chest as well as around vertebrae Nos. 4 to 8 of the spinal column.

**If there is pain on Point No. 36, it means the cause of the trouble is in the heart. Immediately take bed rest for 72 hours** and start taking the following treatment :

( 1 ) Give treatment on Point Nos. 36 and 1 to 5 for two minutes each twice a day.

( 2 ) Give treatment on all the other points on each palm for 5 minutes twice a day.

( 3 ) Drink lukewarm concentrated gold/silver/copper charged water (8 glasses reduced to 2 glasses) 2 glasses a day for 1 month. Thereafter daily 2 glasses reduced from 4 glasses for further 60 days.

( 4 ) Take one pomegranate a day. Either eat it or drink its juice. Just within 30 days, the level of cholesterol will become normal. For prevention, it is advised to eat one pomegranate for 30 days every year.

( 5 ) Practise Pranayam – stop worrying.

During the rest, think over your life style. You will be able to trace the root cause. **Such a root cause must be removed. Otherwise, there can be another heart attack.** Afterwards, lead a normal life, practise Pranayam and do jogging for at least 3 minutes regularly. Continue the treatment on all points and Point No. 36+23 once a day. Drink gold / silver / copper charged water for a month. (8 glasses reduced to 2 glasses)

( 6 ) It has been observed that masturbation in early youth is also one of the root causes of heart attack between the age of 40 to 50. With such previous history, please read the chapter for "Men's Problem" and control sex desire accordingly.

( 7 ) Make a mixture of powders of 100 grams of dried coriander seeds (धनीया) + 100 grams of dried cumin seed (जीरा). Keep it in a bottle. Take 1 teaspoonful of this powder morning and evening for 40 – 50 days. For 30 days take twice a day a mixture of powder of cinamon + honey. This helps in clearing the blockade if any, and prevents operation for byepass surgery. This powder is a good anti-oxidant, also activates liver and thus controls cholestrol.

**Please note that giving two minutes treatment a day on Point No. 36 is like putting a pace maker in the body.**

**Cholesterol :** Reduce fat from diet, drink one glass of fresh juice of pomegranate for 25 to 30 days. **OR** Put 2 teaspoonful of dried coriander (धनीआ) in 4 glasses of water. Boil it and reduce it to 2 glasses. Drink this water daily for 30 days. **OR** Eat powder of dry corriander seeds and cumin seeds. This will bring cholesterol under control.

If any of these juices or drinks is taken for 30 days in a year, it will control cholesterol.

**Case Study 1 :** *Mrs. 'C' aged 75 had to be admitted to the intensive care unit, but she was bored. Her son learnt about Acupressure, brought his mother home and started giving treatment on all the points including Point No. 36 for heart. Today after about four years, she moves freely around the house and is able to look after herself.*

**Case study 2 :** *Mr. 'B' had a heart attack for the second time. In angiography 70% blockade was found in the arteries and so was advised byepass surgery. His sons fixed up the date. Before that I was consulted. I suggested above mentioned treatment. He postponed the operation and followed this treatment very religiously. After 35 days, he again got another angiography and the very same heart specialist declared him to be okay and said that operation was not necessary. Now he is able to live a normal life and he preaches Acupressure.*

In the same way thousands of patients have gone home from intensive care and taken this treatment. Also hundreds of operations for byepass surgery are prevented.

**( 9 ) Diabetes :** Our body requires glucose for energy and so wherever possible take glucose in the natural form, from fruits. its juices, honey, cereals, etc. Moreover this glucose/sugar is easily digestible if it is mixed with saliva. **In order to control diabetes, it is utmost necessary to chew at least 15 times not only eatables but also drinks.** This habit of chewing properly should be formed right from childhood.

Further, instead of adding sugar to the milk make it a practise to drink it plain or add a little turmeric powder that gives milk a good taste and also helps the purification of blood, thus leading to healthy skin.

**Root Causes and their Cure :**

**( 1 ) Tension :** Remove it as per guidelines given on page 221 for nervous tension.

**( 2 ) Pancreas :** In case you find pain on Point No. 25 when pressed, it denotes that this gland is not functioning properly and so enough insulin is not produced to digest the sugar. At that time, if the blood is tested, and found to have 2 % or more, sugar will be found in urine.

For correcting this problem, it is necesary to give treatment on all the endocrine glands. Please note that just by giving this treatment Pancreas can be activated.

**( 3 )** When due to any reason, enough glucose is not extracted from the blood to go into cerebro spinal fluid, the content of glucose in the blood increases. This can be found out by pressing on Point No. 16 of Lymph gland. This can be corrected by drinking daily 2 glasses of charged water reduced from 8 glasses for 30 days and then reduced from 4 glasses for further 30 days and giving treatment on point No. 16. (For more details read author's book "Health in Your Hands : Volume 2")

Moreover, do the following :

( 1 ) Add half a teaspoonful of turmeric powder to one teaspoonful of health drink and take it twice a day for 30 / 45 days.

( 2 ) Cut two lady's fingers (OKRA – भींडी) lengthwise and soak them in half a glass of water overnight. Squeeze them and drink this water the first thing in the morning. If you are susceptible to cold, this squeezed water may be poured on hot pan and drink warm.

**OR**

Drink half a cup of fresh juice of green coriandar leaves हरा धनीया / कोथमीर for 35 – 40 days as the first thing in the morning.

**OR**

Take 8 to 10 mango leaves, soak them in water for half an hour. Then grind the leaves and drink the juice for 35 – 40 days, the first thing in the morning.

After drinking any of the above drinks, you can have regular breakfast after 15 – 20 minutes.

10 to 12 days after you have started this treatment, check up the glucose content in the blood. You will be surprised to find that it is coming down and is under control. Then go on reducing medication for diabetes – pills or insulin injection in such a way as to stop it totally within next ten days. Continue the treatment and just within 30 – 40 days the sugar level will become normal. Continue Acupressure, habit of chewing food and drinking green juice and enjoy the sweet taste and life. Thus this dreaded disease can be easily brought under control.

**Case Study :** *A government officer had 4.5 % glucose in blood. He started drinking the above mentioned juice of green coriander leaves and two glasses of gold/silver/copper charged water along with Acupressure treatment. Within 35 days the glucose level in the blood became normal. Prior to treatment, he was not able to walk. He is now able to walk 4 to 5 miles at a stretch. Thus, he regained his health.*

**Glucosemia :** Many people, for maintaining figure and being afraid of diabetes, go for strict diet control and thus create deficiency of glucose in the body. Another root cause of this disease is overfunctioning of Pancreas which is not understood by other therapies. As many as one out of five Americans may be suffering from this problem. This leads to low B.P., migraine, headache, and even to alcoholism. Life becomes dull and miserable. For cure do the following :

( 1 ) Drink daily two glasses of charged water reduced from four glasses for 30 days. Then daily drink one glass reduced from one and half glasses.

( 2 ) Take more of natural sugar e. g. fruits and honey.

( 3 ) Take treatment on Point No. 25 of Pancreas and all the other endocrine glands, one minute on each point, three times a day.

( 4 ) Drink two cups of green juice adding one teaspoon of health powder one tablespoon of honey to each cup.

Just within 10 to 15 days, this disease will be cured and life will become enjoyable.

**(10) Low Blood Pressure :** Low Blood pressure is due to overfunctioning of Pancreas, thereby reducing the glucose content in the blood and the body. When the blood pressure is low, drinking of hot tea/coffee or milk with more sugar added to it is found effective. For long-term treatment, it is necessary to,

( 1 ) take treatment on all the endocrine glands, along with Acupressure treatment on both the palms/soles.

( 2 ) drink at least two glasses of gold/silver/copper/ iron charged water reduced from 4 glasses of water daily for at least two months.

( 3 ) correct the Solar Plexus if it is not in order.

( 4 ) drink two cups of green juice adding thereto one tablespoonful of honey, one teaspoon of Health drink powder per cup daily.

It may be noted that low B. P. is not dangerous. However, such low B. P. reduces joys of life and makes the life dull. With the above mentioned treatment, life will soon become worth living.

**High Blood Pressure :** The root cause of high B. P. is discussed in the first chapter. As high B. P. leads to many other problems, it is utmost necessary to control it at the earliest. At the time of attack of high B. P. place the small finger in each ear and press them intermittently or shake them hard for 2 to 3 minutes. That will immediately lower the B. P. Also give treatment on Points Nos. 3, 4, 8, 11 to 15, 25 and 28. For long-term cure of this dreaded disease take the following treatment :

( 1 ) Take treatment on all the endocrine glands– 2 minutes on each point – 3 times a day, alongwith regular Acupressure treatment on both the palms/soles.

( 2 ) Drink at least two glasses of gold/silver/copper charged water reduced from four glasses of water. If the use of gold and silver is not possible, drink at least copper+iron charged water two glasses reduced from four glasses of water.

( 3 ) Stop/reduce salt and spices from the diet. Instead rock salt or black salt can be taken.

( 4 ) Drink two cups of green juice adding thereto one tablespoonful of honey + 1 teaspoon of Health Powder per cup.

( 5 ) Drink at least one glass of fruit juice.

( 6 ) Take treatment to reduce tension as shown in this chapter page 221.

Many patients have greatly benefited with the above mentioned treatment and so have stopped taking other treatments.

**(11) Asthma/Breathlessness/Suffocation :** In most of the cases the root cause is "Cold due to heat" and by taking treatment as shown in the previous chapter, this disease can be controlled. In such cases, the lungs would be clear and there will not be any pain on Point No. 30 of lungs.

In case there is pain on Point No. 30, it could be Asthma.

It may be noted that this is a curable disease, the following treatment will be found very effective :

( 1 ) Treatment on Point Nos. 1 to 7, 30, 34 and tips of fingers and toes.

( 2 ) Add $\frac{1}{4}$ teaspoonful of turmeric powder (हलदी) and $\frac{1}{4}$ teaspoonful of powder of cuminseed (जीरा) in one teaspoonful of health drink powder and take it twice a day. If possible, also add $\frac{1}{2}$ teaspoonful of *"Maha-sudarshan"* a bitter powder to the above.

( 3 ) Drink 2 glasses of gold/silver/copper/iron charged water reduced from 8 glasses of water. This is a very effective tonic for lungs.

( 4 ) Take first red light on chest and back, for 2 minutes. Then take blue light for 5 minutes each on chest and back. Do so twice a day.

( 5 ) Perform sun Pranayam as much as possible.

( 6 ) Drink 2 to 3 cups of green juice adding in each cup 1 tablespoon of honey.

( 7 ) Do the following twice a day and also when there is an attack of Asthma.

Press hard on the back, on the points shown in the figure 106 for 10 seconds and pause. Repeat for 2 to 5 minutes.

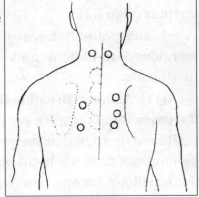

**Fig. 106**

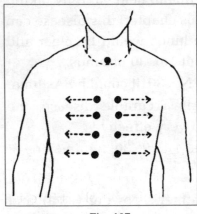

**Fig. 107**

At the same time, ask the patient to rub from the middle of the chest to the sides 2 to 5 minutes. Also give treatment for 1 minute on the point shown below the throat neck. See fig. 107.

These pressing on the back and rubbing on chest are also very useful and effective at the time of an attack of asthma breathlessness.

It may be noted that during this treatment, cold will increase and that is a positive sign of recovery. In that case drink hot/lukewarm water, reduce food/take more of fruits/green juices enabling the body to throw out excess water and toxins from the system.

**Breathlessness :** Press on the points on the back and rub on the chest as shown above. Also do sun Pranayam taking quick short breaths as much as possible. Once you start feeling better finish the Pranayam with prolonged breaths – alternatively from right and left nostril – repeat it at least 10/20 times. Also do Kapalbhati and Bhastrika as mentioned in chapter 5, page 117. It could also be due to blockade in arteries of heart, check Point No. 36 and if it hurts, take treatment as mentioned under (8) of this chapter.

**Eosinophilia :** In cases of continued cold, Asthma, T.B., etc. the percentage of eosinophilia in the blood, is more. In addition to taking the treatment, please take the following treatment for 15 – 20 days.

After sunrise, take half a tablespoonful of half ground Bishop's seeds (अजमा – अजवाईन), soak them in lemon drops for at least 2 hours before eating them, definitely before sunset.

**(12) Rheumatism/Arthritis/Paralysis/Stroke :** Frequent colds, mostly due to excess heat in the body or improper digestion, damage the working of Thyroid and parathyroid glands leading to inadequate digestion of calcium in the body. This in turn damages the working of Gonads/Sex glands which control the digestion of phosphorus. The combined effect is that the internal heat of the body reduces giving way to water level in the body to increase. Now, when the internal heat of the body is reduced in old age or due to weakness or continuous cold, there is pain in small joints called "Rheumatic Arthritis". Sometimes there is swelling in big joints and if not cured, it has a bad effect on the heart and so it is called "Rheumatoid Arthritis". When these problems of joint pains are tried to be suppressed by more and more powerful drugs, it impairs the nervous system. Moreover, damage to Thyroid, Parathyroid and Sex glands leads to damage to Adrenal gland which causes less oxygenation in the body. **As a result of all these plus tension leads to stroke/paralysis.**

Now, when we know the root causes of this painful chronic disease, it can be easily prevented by taking treatment on all endocrine glands and curing the cold in the beginning by understanding its root cause.

**Treatment :** This disease can be cured by the following treatment :

( 1 ) Take treatment on all points of both the palms, five minutes on each palm twice a day.

( 2 ) Roll the soles on wooden rollers five minutes – twice a day. See fig. 69.

( 3 ) Take treatment on all the endocrine glands 2/2 minutes on each point twice a day.

( 4 ) Drink 2 glasses of gold/silver/copper charged water reduced from 8 glasses of water, lukewarm if possible.

( 5 ) Rub nylon brush (big one used for washing clothes) on each sole 5 minutes in the morning and 5 minutes in the evening till the soles get warmer than the head.

( 6 ) Take half a teaspoonful of *Mahasudarshan* powder +half a teaspoonful of turmeric powder with water once in morning and once in evening. Avoid sour things totally from the diet.

( 7 ) (a) Make a mixture of
Calc. Phos 200–
+Calc. Fl. – 200–
+Nat. Mur– 200–
+Fer. Phos– 200–
$\left.\right\}$ $\frac{1}{2}$ oz each

and take 4 pills in the morning and 4 pills in the evening for 10 days and then once a week.

(b) Make a mixture of
Calc. Phos
Calc. Fl.
Nat. Mur
Fer. Phos
$\left.\right\}$ $12 \times \frac{1}{2}$ oz each

After 10 days take daily 4 pills in the morning +4 pills in evening for two months.

( 8 ) Take red light on the affected area (not head) for 4 to 5 minutes on each part. Then take blue light for 5 to 6 minutes on each affected part + on head also. Take this light twice daily till the disease is cured.

In such cases rolling of feet for 5 minutes on wooden roller shown in fig. 108 has been found beneficial.

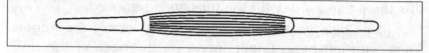

**Fig. 108 (See fig. 69 on page 125)**

[**Note :** It may be noted that effect of such plain cheap wooden roller is just the same as that of costly fancy rollers.]

*Mr. 'G' had an attack of paralysis. He found that the points of thyroid/parathyroid and adrenal glands were paining. He started the treatment as above and just within 12 days, he became normal.*

**Gout :** The same treatment as mentioned above for asthma is found to be useful. Moreover, take 1 tablespoonful of castor oil alongwith 1 teaspoonful of ginger powder at least twice a week till complete cure is achieved.

**(13) Nervous Tension :** In the modern days because of fast life and loss of contentment, nervous tension keeps on building up increasingly, tending to damage our mind and health.

**How to find out :** Ask the patient to lie down on the back and ask some one to press on the base of the middle toe in both the legs. If there is a hurting sensation, it means nervous

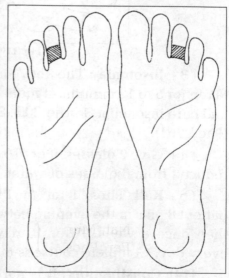

**Fig. 109**

tension. If the hurting is unbearable, it means that the person is on the verge of collapse and needs immediate attention. See fig. 109.

**Cure :** ( 1 ) While the patient is lying on the back, bend all the toes of both legs, backward. It may hurt but give little more pressure and bend them as much as possible. Repeat this three times a day till the tension is removed.

( 2 ) Clasp your hands tightly interlocking the fingers. Then with left hand fingers press on the back of the right hand and then with right hand fingers, press on the back of the left hand. Repeat for about 1 to 2 minutes, 3 to 4 times a day. See fig. 110.

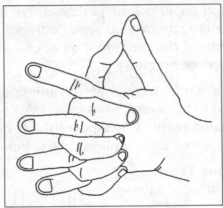

**Fig. 110**

( 3 ) **Insomnia :** The above mentioned treatment can be taken for 5 to 12 minutes at night in bed to ensure good sleep and cure insomnia. See fig. 110. Sometimes, salt can be used (Page 264).

( 4 ) Give 2 glasses of gold/silver/copper charged water reduced from 8 glasses of water.

( 5 ) **Kali Phos 1 m (a Biochemic medicine) :** Give patient 8 pills in the evening between 8 to 9 p. m. for 10 days, then once a week. After 10 days Kali Phos 12 × 4 + 4 pills every day. Complete course is of 45 days.

**(14) Constipation :** It is not necessary to take laxative. Acupressure treatment plus drinking of lukewarm water and giving the stomach some rest at least of one meal during a week will set the things right. Also include more water/buttermilk and leafy vegetables in the diet.

First check the Solar Plexus and if not in order correct it as shown on page 73. Put the thumb on the middle of chin (see fig. 111) and rub it or give pressure around it for 2 to 6 minutes. This will solve the problems of constipation. An essential requirement of health is that there should be no constipation.

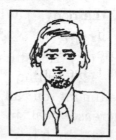

Fig. 111

If it is felt that passing of stools is not satisfactory, wet the middle long finger with coconut oil/edible oil or butter and put it as far as possible in the anus and massage around it. Afterwards, move the belly, inwards and out. Further stools may start coming out. Clean the part with water. This treatment helps to clean the bowels, prevent constipation and also the piles. **Moreover, as there is massage around prostate gland, it activates the same and problems of prostate gland, hernia, frequent urination, etc. are also cured. This is called "Ganesh Kriya" in yoga.**

**(15) Piles/Fissures :** These are caused by continuous constipation. Some times piles not only give severe pain but also start bleeding. For treatment, first remove constipation as mentioned above. Also give treatment on Point No. 10 on both the palms or soles. Also massage coconut oil or castor oil on piles. Do "Ganesh Kriya".

*Mr. 'K' had piles which had started bleeding. He started treatment under this therapy by applying pressure on Point No. 10, 3 times a day. Within 2 days his bleeding stopped and within 8 days the complaint was gone.*

**(16) Obesity :** This is due to :

( 1 ) Malfunctioning of Thyroid/Parathyroid gland and later on other endocrine glands e. g. malfunctioning of Pineal gland leads to retention of water and excess water in the body and leads to excess fat.

( 2 ) Underworking of Sex glands mainly in ladies after delivery of a child.

( 3 ) Overeating i. e. taking more calories than required by the body.

**Cure :**

( 1 ) Take treatment on all endocrine glands twice daily.

( 2 ) During pregnancy and after delivery, take treatment on all the endocrine glands. After delivery, increase heat in the body as mentioned on page 262 (1) (a), (b), (c).

( 3 ) Drink charged water daily two glasses reduced from 4 glasses.

( 4 ) Drink hot to lukewarm water only during the day and always after meals.

( 5 ) In the morning in one glass of hot water add juice of half a lemon and one tablespoonful of honey. Drink it That will reduce the desire to eat/drink sweets.

( 6 ) Chew food at least 15 times.

( 7 ) Drink 3 to 5 cups of green juice a day adding 1 teaspoonful of health drink to each cup. This will help to reduce the body very fast without any side effects and make the skin fresh. Do not throw away the waste. Add little cream of milk and turmeric powder and apply it on the face as mask. Also take blue light on the face for 5 minutes. Wash the face after 15/20 minutes. You will be surprised to see the result in 15/20 days. Wrinkle and spots will vanish and the colour of skin will become fair and shining.

( 8 ) Eat plenty of salads adding 100 grams of sprouted cereals like Mung (मूंग). Also eat two seasonal fruits + 1 glass of buttermilk.

( 9 ) Avoid all food if possible. However, in spite of the above diet, if you feel very hungry, take preparations of only wheat or only rice. That will reduce the intake of food. But eat this food only when you are very hungry.

(10) Do Pranayam + Ling Mudra + Acupressure

**Case Study :** *One obese lady started the above mentioned treatment religiously–she stopped all food. For energy, she would take two tablespoonful of honey in a day. Within 30 days, she lost 10 Kgs, continued treatment for further 60 days and lost total 22 Kgs. Her skin became smooth and shining. She continued Acupressure. Even after five years, she has maintained her normal weight of 62 Kgs and won back the love of her husband.*

Sugar and fat can be reduced and controlled. To reduce weight, diet has to be very strictly regulated. Sugar, sweets, oil and butter–ghee in any form should be totally stopped and salt to be reduced to the minimum or only rock salt should be taken. Secondly, the diet should include plenty of vegetables, green juices, a few fruits, sprouted pulses and wheat products. Rice and its different preparations should be avoided or if the diet includes rice and its preparations wheat, jowar, bajra, etc., should be avoided. This will enable the patient to restrict the quantity of food intake and fat will start reducing. In short, the intake of food should be brought down to below 900 calories. During the dieting, the patient, should drink lukewarm health drink or lemon water and honey, the first thing in the morning. Then during the day he should drink boiled lukewarm water only, preferably copper/silver/gold charged. He should also drink four cups of green juice a day.

**How to control Hunger and reduce Weight :** In order that hunger itself be reduced, please give deeper pressure on the three points in the ears half an hour before the meals as shown in fig. 112.

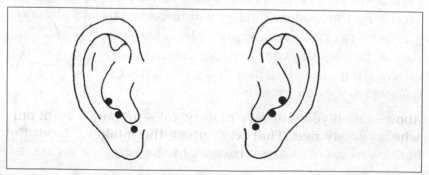

**Fig. 112**

Pressure can be given by keeping the thumb behind the ear and giving deeper pressure by fingers. In order to get better results, avoid sweets, ice-cream, fried things and rice from diet and have more of green vegetables and juice and fruits. Drink at least 4 glasses of gold/silver charged water duly reduced from 10 glasses of water.

Practise sun Pranayam daily for 15 – 20 minutes and start taking light exercise, longer walks, etc. If possible, massage the body with oil at least twice a week.

Once the weight is brought down, regular Acupressure treatment will help you to maintain your proper weight.

**(17) How to stop Bad Habits :** Most of the people are aware of the harmful effects of their bad habits like smoking, drinking alcohol, chewing of tobacco, overeating, etc. In spite of their desire to give up such habits, they are not able to do so for lack of the necessary will-power.

Acupressure can greatly help people to cure themselves of their bad habits. Give treatment on all the points specially on all the points of the endocrine glands twice a day. After 15 days, you will get the necessary will-power to stop these bad habits. On the 16th day, you take a vow to stop the bad habit. Continue this treatment to prevent any side effects on the body.

The following treatment will be found useful in specific problems :

**(A) Smoking and Chewing of Tobacco :**

( 1 ) During the 15 days when Acupressure treatment is taken as above, give pressure on the 2 points of both the ears as shown in the figure. This pressure is to be given as many times as possible. This will control the desire to smoke and the quantum of smoking or chewing tobacco will be reduced to a great extent.

( 2 ) Pranayam as shown in this book is a must and may be practised as many times as possible. That will give strength to the tired lungs.

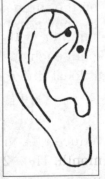

Fig. 113

### (B) Alcoholism :

( 1 ) Please check up your Pancreas gland. If it is over-working, you will have more and more desire to drink. It is therefore necessary to control this gland by the treatment mentioned above for giving up bad habits.

( 2 ) Cultivate the habit of drinking hot water in the evening or whenever there is a desire to drink alcohol.

( 3 ) Rub the tip of nose for 2 minutes twice a day (see fig. 114). This treatment is also useful in case of drunkenness. The person will become sober instantly. It is possible that he may vomit; so the person giving this treatment should remain by the side and not in front of the drunken person.

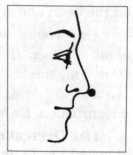

Fig. 114

*Mr. 'X' used to take a minimum of 3 pegs in the evening. He started this treatment and began drinking half a glass of hot water. Within 15 days he was satisfied with one peg only. Later on, he stopped drinking.*

### (C) Drug Addiction :

( 1 ) Continue the treatment for 2 / 2 minutes three times a day on the point shown in the figure on both the sides of head. See fig. 115.

( 2 ) Give general treatment together with 2/2 minutes treat-ment each on the endocrine glands at least thrice a day.

( 3 ) Give 2 glasses of gold/ silver/copper charged water reduced from 6 glasses for one month. Then 2 glasses of this water reduced from 4 glasses for a further period of 2 months.

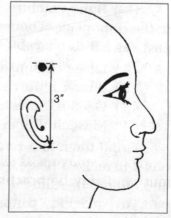

Fig. 115

( 4 ) Desire for drugs will be greatly reduced within 15-20 days. Then only can the patient be asked to stop the drugs. Meanwhile the quantity of drug may be reduced progressively.

( 5 ) Give the patient 2 to 3 cups of green juices and 1 to 2 glasses of fruit juice.

( 6 ) During the treatment for 3 months, give blue light on the head and spinal cord for 5 minutes each twice a day.

*One young man aged 22, had been taking drugs for about 6 years. He had also the habit of masturbation. He started the treatment. After 20 days, he stopped taking drugs. Within 45 days, he was also cured of the habit of masturbation. He became an ardent follower of Acupressure.*

**(D) Overeating :** Chew your food and drink thoroughly at least 12 to 15 times before gulping down. Observe silence while eating. Stop eating at the second signal you get from the stomach. If necessary, make a habit of taking food after every 4 hours but do not overeat at a time. Control the endocrine glands.

**(18) Burns :** Massage the point on both the hands as shown in the figure strongly and burning sensation will be reduced considerably.

**(19) Bone Fracture :** First set the bone in the right place. Then apply the following paste as hot as bearable :

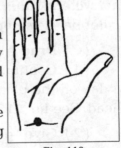

Fig. 116

( 1 ) Litsea chinenses (Menda Lakadi)  100 grams
( 2 ) Rhubarb (Reva chini)  50 grams
( 3 ) Gelatin (Saresh)  50 grams
( 4 ) Mastich (Ruma Mastaki)  4 grams

Grind them to a powder. Mix the powder in water and boil it to make a paste. Apply the paste on the fractured part and around it. Allow it to dry. Give support to the affected part by placing cotton over it and covering it with a cardboard or stick and then bandage it.

Next day, clean this paste with lukewarm water and Dettol. Then again apply this paste in the above mentioned way. Repeat this process for 8 days. During this period, give treatment on the tips of fingers and toes of the affected side of the body. Also drink 2 glasses of charged water reduced from 4 glasses of water.

This treatment is used by the people living in the Marwar desert and it is found to be very effective by bonesetters. *A leading bonesetter in Mumbai reports : "After properly setting the fractured bones, I give this treatment for all types of single and multiple fractures and within 8 to 10 days the patients get cured."*

**(20) Elephantiasis (Filariasis) :**

( 1 ) Roll your feet on the grooved wooden roller for five minutes in the morning and in the evening.

( 2 ) Roll the grooved wooden roller on the affected part for 5 minutes twice a day. (See fig. 108)

( 3 ) Drink silver charged water 2 glasses reduced from 6 glasses twice a day.

( 4 ) Afterwards take treatment on all points daily especially on the points relating to kidneys–for 2 minutes three times a day.

( 5 ) Drink black tea as per page 187 for 15 days.

( 6 ) Drink daily 2 to 4 cups of green juice adding thereto 1 teaspoon of health powder.

( 7 ) One can also apply afterwards, remaining paste of green juice on affected area as mentioned on page 169 – 170.

**(21) Leprosy/Leukoderma (White Spots) :**

( 1 ) The reason for Leprosy is excess heat and non-perspiration through certain parts of the skin and less functioning of liver.

( 2 ) As more and more toxins gather under that part of skin, the nerves ending at that place become dead and numbness is found on that particular part of the skin and the colour of the patch changes to white.

( 3 ) When this is not treated at the right time and when proper nourishment is not taken or when the Adrenal glands are not functioning properly, the other ends of the nerves situated in the hands or feet get affected and their deterioration starts.

( 4 ) Later on when lymph glands work less, these affected parts of the hands and feet become septic and pus starts oozing out and then other parts of the body, especially nose, etc., are also affected.

**To cure leprosy :**

( 1 ) Treatment should be taken on points of liver, gall bladder and Adrenal glands and other glands to ensure proper oxygenation and blood circulation.

( 2 ) **Treatment is to be given on the point of kidneys to throw out the toxins from the body.** And also drink black tea for 15/20 days; as mentioned under Pyelitis in chapter 14 under (22) page 187.

( 3 ) On the numb parts of the skin, ice is to be rubbed for 3 to 5 minutes and then heated self-urine or any healthy person's or cow's urine, after taking out the crust, should be rubbed on the affected part and around it with cotton wool for five minutes in the morning and evening and then the parts should be washed with lukewarm water.

( 4 ) Sunbath is to be given on the affected parts twice a day for 10 to 15 minutes. If sunbath is not possible, blue light should be given to the affected parts for 7 to 10 minutes.

( 5 ) Charged silver/copper water (two glasses reduced from eight glasses) should be given to the patient to drink.

( 6 ) Intake of salt should be totally stopped or if necessary rock salt may be given.

( 7 ) Drink 3 to 4 cups of green juice. Also apply green paste.

( 8 ) Make a mixture of whole wheat flour, gram flour and turpentine; apply it on the affected parts twice a day and keep it for 15 minutes. If the skin becomes dry and is stretched, rub a little coconut oil on and around the affected parts. Afterwards, apply green paste and take blue light.

**(22) Gangrene :** If the patient is not diabetic, get his first urine in the morning, otherwise, first urine of a healthy person or even that of a cow can be used.

Boil this urine and allow it to cool. Remove the crust from the urine.

In case, gangrene is in the leg, apply ice manufactured out of ammonia (not from the fridge) and apply it from hips to toes especially on all joints for 3 to 5 minutes. Afterwards, massage the above mentioned warm urine with cotton on all the parts from hips to toes, and rub this warm urine for 5 to 7 minutes on the affected parts. Cover the affected part with cotton and bandage it. After 2 hours, clean the affected part with dettol, savlon or any antiseptic. Repeat the same treatment in the evening. Within 2 to 5 days, the affected parts will dry up and gangrene will be cured.

In the same way, in the case of gangrene is on the back apply ice from the starting point of the spinal cord up to the thighs, especially on all the joints and then apply warm urine on all the parts and especially massage the affected part with urine for 5 to 7 minutes.

Also take treatment on Point No. 16, lymph gland for 2 minutes, 3 times a day and drink 2 glasses of charged water reduced from 6 glasses.

**(23) Syphilis and other Venereal Diseases :** (1) Massage ice on the affected part for 2 to 4 minutes. (2) If the patient is not diabetic, take his first urine and add 1–2 teaspoons of soda-bicarb to it, boil the urine and allow to cool. Remove the upper crust and with cotton soaked in the urine, massage the affected part and around it for 5 to 7 minutes. Afterwards, clean the affected part with water containing dettol or any other antiseptic. Bandage the affected part.

Continue this treatment twice a day for 3 to 4 days. Also take the treatment for the control of sex desire as mentioned in chapter 12, page 160, Fig. no. 80.

**(24) Cancer :** It is a man-made dreaded disease. The main point of worry in the case of cancer is that when it is detected, it has already reached an advanced stage and the possibility of complete cure is remote. Moreover, the treatment is so costly that the patient and his/her relatives get financially and mentally exhausted.

The immediate cause for cancer is the continuous neglect of the organs of the body by the patient. For example, the lungs of a chain-smoker are continuously irritated. The cancer of the mouth or vocal cords is due to the habit of chewing tobacco, drinking hot tea, etc. In the case of cancer of the uterus, negligence about internal hygiene is the root cause. It has been observed that Jewish women who take great care of their internal organs, do not get cancer of the uterus.

Cancer of the breast is due to non-feeding of the baby by mother, and suppression of the sexual desire by unmarried women.

Cancer of the stomach and intestines is due to overuse of refined flour and rice, coffee, sugar and tea and the habit of overdrinking of alcohol. It has been observed that labourers in the sugar factory in the West Indies use brown sugar molasses–jaggery and so they are immune to cancer. **And cancer of colon is due to continuous constipation caused by wrongful habits of food and sedentary life.** It has been observed that the people of Gujarat who are vegetarian and use more of milk and milk products like curd, buttermilk, etc., do not generally get this type of cancer.

Another reason is a wrongful approach towards the body. The diseases are nothing but the signals given by the body that there is something wrong in that organ, e. g. tonsils.

Instead of removing the root cause of the disease, either the signal, tonsils or appendix is removed by operation or the disease is suppressed like common cold with powerful antibiotics. The body is to be treated as a temple – a seat of God and each and every corner of this temple, body, should be kept neat and clean. Instead, the body is treated like a dustbin wherein useless things are dumped and instead of cleaning out the waste or toxins, they are suppressed; with the result it becomes a duct and which after a time results into a malignant growth.

The long-term cause of cancer is the imbalance caused by disturbing the metabolism of the body through (1) eatables grown with the help of inorganic manure and pesticides, (2) more and more use of canned foods, bottled pickles, (3) unwise use of fluoride (4) working in unhygienic conditions e. g. working in asbestos factory and smoking, (5) pollution of the environment by excessive use of diesel, cutting down of trees, etc. (6) polluting the water through chemical wastes, etc. (7) going farther and farther away from Nature.

It will, thus, be observed that these root causes of cancer can be removed and thus cancer can be prevented. You will find that in the animal world this dreaded disease is rarely found. The obvious reason is that they follow laws of Nature.

**How cancer develops :** In our body millions of new cells are formed every day and they replace the old worn out cells. This process is carried out by the spleen and it is cleaned and controlled by the Lymph glands. When we neglect our body, the process of regeneration of new cells slows down while the process of decaying-destroying of cells-increases, more toxins gather in the body, the spleen and Lymph glands are overburdened. Slowly but steadily, there is a malignant growth in the body, but it is not easily noticed. Meanwhile, these toxins/wastes gather in the body in the part which is most damaged e. g. for a smoker, these toxins gather in the lungs or in the mouth. When these toxins are gathered in a large quantity, it forms a duct and starts developing fast. In the meantime, the weak Lymph gland is greatly damaged and through it other glands are damaged. And a stage is reached when these glands become tired and stop secreting the most vital hormones in the body. At that time, this malignant growth becomes fast and the final signal is given by Nature. There is a change in metabolism, severe headache, loss of weight, change of voice, colour of the spots on the body changes, and constant fever. At this time, this disease is diagnosed as cancer.

**Acupressure plays a great role in the detection, prevention and cure of cancer.**

Any minor disturbance of any organ is reflected on the palms or soles. When there is a continued complaint the first gland to be disturbed is the Thyroid/Parathyroid gland. The second gland to be disturbed in case of problems of degeneration leading towards cancer is the Lymph gland. As mentioned above, this important gland works to remove the toxins and dead cells from the body. When the process of regeneration of the cells of the body slows down, there is increase in the activity of clearing the dead cells and preventing pus formation. This gland, thus, gives ALARM. If you touch on its Point No. 16, on hands and feet, these points are found to be tender and when you press them, you will feel pain.

**How to detect Cancer in different parts of body.**

Another pointer for detection is that the organ where cancer is developing is disturbed and there is pain in the corresponding point on palms and soles. For example, in case of cancer of the breast, there is pain in the middle point on the back of palm as shown in fig. 118 or in case of cancer of colon, there is pain in Point No. 20.

The same way, for cancer in

| | |
|---|---|
| Throat | : There is pain on Point No. 6 |
| Windpipe gullet | : There is pain between point No. 6 and 27 |
| Stomach | : There is pain on Point No. 27 |
| Small Intestine | : There is pain on Point No. 19 |
| Large Intestine & Colon | : There is pain on Point No. 20 and 10 |
| Liver | : Point No. 23 and 22 |
| Lungs | : Point No. 30 |
| Brain | : Point Nos. 1 to 5 (It is also called tumour) |
| Blood | : Point No. 37 |
| Bones | : Point Nos. 9 & 37 |

Now, if these signals are ignored, the declining process starts disturbing other glands also and reaches a dangerous point where these endocrine glands become tired and stop secreting hormones. During that time, more and more wastes/toxins accumulate forming a duct and start multiplying and thus a fast malignant growth starts in that part of the body damaging the very metabolism of the body.

Thus, you will observe that cancer can be detected at a very early stage, and it can be controlled very easily. Moreover, you will observe that if regular Acupressure treatment is taken daily or at least 3 times a week the lethargic spleen or lymph gland can be reactivated, and factors leading to cancer can be checked. **Thus Acupressure can prevent Cancer.**

**How to detect cancer of the uterus :** It is more common in ladies who do not take proper care of internal hygeine. It is due to continuous irregularity of menstruation, continuous Leucorrhoea etc. This type of cancer can be easily detected. In case of any doubt, press on Point Nos. 11 to 15 on both the sides of wrists of both the hands. If there is pain on pressing these points and also on Point No. 16 of lymph gland, it denotes degeneration.

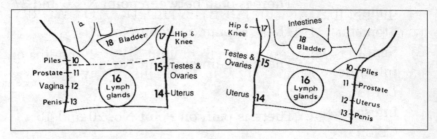

Fig. 117

**How to detect cancer of breasts mamography :** Just press on the circle in the back of the right palm for right breast and left palm for left breast. If, there is NO PAIN when pressed; it means there is NO CANCER in the breasts. Even if, there is pain on these points, but no pain on Point No. 16 of Lymph gland at that time, it denotes that there is NO CANCER. And just by giving treatment on those

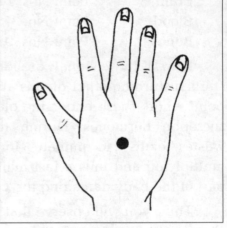

Fig. 118

points on the back of palms, the minor problem like accumulation of milk in the breast, etc. will be cured. Only pain on the circles on the back of right palm and also on the Point No. 16 of Lymph gland; denotes cancer degeneration in the right breast. In the same way, cancer in the left breast can be detected by pressing the circle on the back of left palm and Point No. 16 of Lymph gland.

At that time, it is possible that when pressed, there will be pain on Point Nos. 11 to 15 of the sex glands.

Severe pain on those points on the back side of palms and on Point No. 16 when pressed, denotes that cancer has developed more.

EVEN IF, CANCER IS DETECTED, DO NOT WORRY. IT IS EASILY CURABLE.

**Cure :** Give Acupressure treatment for 2 – 2 minutes on each of the following points for three times a day :

( 1 ) On the circles on the back of palms, for cancer of the breasts. See fig. 118.

( 2 ) On Point Nos. 11 to 15 on both sides of the wrists for cancer of the uterus. See fig. 117.

( 3 ) On Point No. 16 on both the hands.

( 4 ) On points of all the endocrine glands i. e. Nos. 3, 4, 8, 25 and 28.

( 5 ) Take general Acupressure treatment on all the points twice a day. And on Point No. 26 as a last treatment.

( 6 ) Drink 'black tea' one cup in the early morning (see page 187).

( 7 ) The use of vaginal douche is a must for the treatment of cancer of the uterus and the breasts.

First clean the douche with water containing antiseptic. Take about 1 litre of lukewarm water and add 2 to 4 drops of antiseptic liquid to it. Then fill the douche with this water by pressing the ball. Then keep the plastic part (2 inches) into vagina and press the ball.

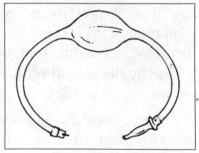

Fig. 119 : Vaginal Douche

Water will flow inside and clean it. Repeat it for 2 / 4 times. Such use of Vaginal Douche is also useful when pus cells are found in the urine of a lady i. e. in case of infection in Urine.

( 8 ) Make the necessary change in diet as mentioned for the treatment of cancer.

(9) In case of more pain on the points on the back of palms and Point No. 16 and also when lumps are found in the breasts, apply North Pole of a (low to medium power) magnet on the lumps only for 3/5 minutes 2 to 3 times a day.

*"A lady of 50 years was found to have cancer in both the breasts and was advised operation. Instead she took the above treatment and was completely cured within 45 days."*

*"A 40 year old lady, a mother of 4 children, was found to have cancer of the uterus. Cancer was detected even in her left breast. She started the above mentioned Acupressure treatment and continued the same for 60 days. Later on, her husband came and thanked me saying that he got a 'New Wife'– 10 years younger. In the same way several cases have been successfully treated."*

It is observed that in more than two hundred cases where dialysis was being done and when proper improvement was not found, these patients were advised to undergo transplantation of kidney. In all these cases, on examination, damage to kidney was not more than 40 to 50 % – and the root cause was found to be cancer of the uterus in females and that of prostate in males. Within 40 to 60 days of Acupressure treatment all the patients got cured. It is, therefore, advisable that before undergoing dialysis and transplantation of kidney to check up about the possibility of cancer.

It has been also agreed by the Medical World that if cancer is detected at an early stage, it can be cured.

**Cure for all types of cancer :** To cure all types of cancer the whole body is to be treated, the important organs of regeneration e. g. liver, gall bladder, spleen and kidneys and all the endocrine glands are to be reactivated. Acupressure treatment assists the patient in the process and accelerates recovery by bringing the metabolism of the body in order.

Following treatments are suggested :

( 1 ) Check up the Solar Plexus and put it in order.

( 2 ) Banish salt and spices from the diet.

( 3 ) For ten days, take an enema of water boiled with coffee twice a day. That helps to open up the ducts and remove the toxins from the body. Afterwards, take the enema three times a week for further four weeks.

( 4 ) In case ducts / lumps have developed, take vapour treatment (as mentioned on page 132), on the ducts and cold packs treatment in the case of cancer of the stomach and uterus page 202. Also apply north pole of magnet on the ducts for 3/5 minutes 2 times a day. It will dissolve the duct.

( 5 ) Take concentrated lukewarm water of copper, silver and gold, 3 to 4 glasses, during the day. Boil 20 glasses of water and reduce it to 4 glasses.

( 6 ) In diet, have only fresh juices of vegetables as mentioned on page 169 and of fruits like grapes, pomegranate, etc. In the diet, juice of sprouted pulses, beet root, carrot and cabbage should be included. Such a diet helps the patient to gain weight. Eat plenty of salads and honey.

( 7 ) Take Acupressure treatment on all the points twice a day. Also give special extra treatment of 2 minutes on each point of endocrine glands – Point Nos. 3, 4, 8, 14, 15, 16, 25, 28 and 38 (in case of children). After the treatment is taken, take treatment on Point No. 26 of kidneys also.

( 8 ) Practise Pranayam regularly as often as possible.

( 9 ) Take sunbath and if it is not possible, take blue light on the affected part of the body for 8 to 10 minutes.

(10) In case of cancer in the mouth, throat and gullet :

( a ) First cure Pyorrhoea, if it is there. If the condition of teeth is bad and the Dentist advises removal of them, please get such teeth removed.

( b ) Take 5 drops of Glycerine Acid Tanic (available in chemist's shop); add little quantity of turmeric powder to the same. Apply this paste on both the sides inside the throat.

Then, gargle with salted lukewarm water. Do this twice/thrice a day.

( c ) On an empty stomach in the morning, ask the patient to lie down on the back and open his mouth wide open. Then, pour 1 table spoonful of honey in such a way that this honey does not touch the tongue. Repeat this in the afternoon but definitely before sunset.

(11) For the first 10/15 days, drink pineapple juice as shown below :

Take a ripe pineapple, cut it into two halves horizontally, squeeze the juice of the half and drink it the first thing in the morning and drink the juice of the balance half in the evening before sunset. If desired, honey can be added to the juice. This fresh juice of pineapple creates a cooling effect and removes excess heat. It has got such a therapeutic value that it cures cancer of gullet, stomach, liver and intestines.

(12) Drink the extract of the following the first thing in the morning (even before you take pineapple juice).

21 Leaves of bitter neem with stalk.

21 Leaves of tulsi with stalk.

21 Leaves of bilipatra (7 × 3) with stalk.

This is a MUST in case of cancer of blood, bones, and brain and wherever to be used as a blood purifier.

(Only if such leaves are not available, tincture of the same is available at Homeopathic medicine shops. Take 5 drops in half a cup of lukewarm water in the morning and evening.)

(13) After 12 to 15 days or when, the patient gets very hungry (it is a good sign of recovery), give the patient 3 to 4 ounces of curd, prepared in the following manner. To the boiled warm milk (preferebly of cow's or goat's milk) add 12/15 leaves of tulsi and prepare the curd. If the patient is of Pitt Prakruti, give him this curd, adding thereto little powder of crystal sugar. For all other types of patients, this

curd can be taken with little rock salt or black salt in it. Such curd can be taken 3 to 4 times a day. from 10 a.m. to 5 p.m. only.

(14) Eat roasted bitter gourd (Karela-कारेला) as mentioned on page 194. Treatment mentioned especially in 11 to 14 has been found effective even in blood cancer.

(15) Give the following combination of biochemic powder/pills :

| | | |
|---|---|---|
| Calc. Phos | 30 × | 1 oz |
| Kali Phos | 30 × | 1 oz |
| Kali Muir | 30 × | 1 oz |
| Ferrum Phos | 30 × | 1 oz |
| Kali Iodide | 30 × | 1 oz |

(If Kali Iodide is not available in powder/pills, add its tincture to other pills/powder) Give 2 grains powder or 6 pills – 3 times a day. After taking this medicine, do not take anything for 10/15 minutes.

(16) **In case any or more endocrine glands are severely damaged, e. g. hypothyroid, etc., the above treatment is necessary.**

(17) We should not forget that cancer is the last warning of nature. Go back to nature and within a short period, you will be able to control and cure this dreaded disease. **It is likely that during the first 8 to 12 days, the patient may have nausea, vomitting or severe headache. He/She may refuse to take enema, etc. But continue the treatment.** Improvement will be observed within 15 to 20 days, and complete cure within 45 to 90 days depending upon the stage of cancer when this treatment is started. **Even if the development of cancer is more than 85 % and is not curable, this treatment will be helpful.** The unbearable pain will definitely subside and death will be peaceful.

(18) After recovery, take a balanced diet consisting of 50 to 60 % whole wheat and cereals, plus vegetables and milk products. Avoid salt. If desired, use rock salt or black salt.

It has been noticed that people in Gujarat who have this type of diet do not get cancer of the stomach or intestine.

(19) This dreaded, disease results from utter neglect and undue harassment of the body and our bad habits in the past life. Accept the result calmly, forgive all, pray to God and take a vow to do only good deeds, to be of some help to others after recovery. **Please note that prayers have more power than drugs. And last but not the least, have self-confidence and be cheerful.**

(20) Get rid of bad habits as already shown in this book on page 226.

(21) If Allopathic drugs are taken, take Thuja 200 – 4 pills for 3 days. If rays are taken, take treatment to remove excess heat as mentioned under useful hints. 2 (a) & (b) on page 262.

**The following are forbidden :**

Processed and canned foods, salted pickle, frozen, jarred, bleached or refined foods, also coffee, tea, tobacco, alcohol, spices, salt, hair dyes, pain relieving agents and drugs, fluorinated water and toothpaste, and temporarily (till the liver starts functioning well), cheese, eggs, fish, meat and milk.

To eradicate this dreaded disease from this world, its root causes namely, pollution of air, pollution of wheat, rice, barley, maize etc, staple food, through inorganic manure and over-use of insecticides, excessive use of preservatives in canned and bottled fruits and food products, excessive use of tobacco, alcohol, sugar and coffee, meat etc., must be avoided. This can be done by the World Health Organization and U.N.O. But meanwhile, people can take care of themselves and prevent these root causes in their own interest, and with the help of Acupressure, can give up their bad habits, and thus prevent this dreaded disease of cancer.

**All types of cancer, including that of blood, are successfully treated. Even patients, discharged from cancer hospital, as incurable, were eventually cured with the above**

mentioned treatment, given to them by their relatives in their homes and that too without any costs. Several such cases can be quoted;

**Case Study :**

( 1 ) Mr. "A" was discharged from cancer hospital as his cancer of throat was considered incurable. He was in such agony that painkiller injections had to be given 3 times a day. On the fifth day of treatment, painkiller injections were no more required. On the sixteenth day, he started getting good hunger and within 45 days only, he was totally cured and resumed normal duties.

( 2 ) Mrs. "M" the wife of an M. D. Doctor tried several therapies for her loss of weight and failing stamina. At last an Acupressurist was consulted. He diagnosed the problems as cancer of stomach. Treatment was started at home with the permission of her husband. Within 60 days, she got cured, gained weight and stamina. Now, she propagates Acupressure.

( 3 ) A college student, 19 years old, was so much disturbed with his problem that he started thinking of committing suicide. An Acupressurist was consulted. He diagnosed it as a case of cancer of the prostate. Without knowing any previous history, he told the young man that he was in a practice of masturbation for a long time. The boy admitted it. With a treatment of only 40 days, the boy was cured. Now he intends to be a Professor. He himself has become an ardent Acupressurist and confidently treats patients.

**(25) Thalasemmia :** It is a dreaded disease found in children. In acute cases, total blood has to be transfused every 15 to 30 days. In spite of best treatment and blood transfusion, chances of recovery are very limited. **On examination of such patients, it has been found that their endocrine glands are severely damaged and even all organs of digestive system are found to be sluggish.**

The treatment as mentioned above for cancer of blood is found very useful and effective. **At the same time, for the deficiency of haemoglobin in their blood (the same way for all patients of severe anaemia)** the following treatment along with the medicines for anaemia as mentioned on page 156 will give astonishing results.

**Treatment for increasing haemoglobin :** Take black dried raisins as may be required daily. Soak them in half a cup of water overnight. Eat these black raisins as mentioned below and drink the water.

|  | Morning | Afternoon | Evening |
|---|---|---|---|
| 1st day | 1 | 1 | 1 |
| 2nd day | 2 | 2 | 2 |
| 3rd day | 3 | 3 | 3 |
| 4th day | 4 | 4 | 4 |
| 5th day | 4 | 4 | 4 |
| 6th day | 4 | 4 | 4 |
| 7th day | 3 | 3 | 3 |
| 8th day | 2 | 2 | 2 |
| 9th day | 1 | 1 | 1 |

Check the haemoglobin level of the blood. If necessary, repeat as above after 8/10 days and continue in the same way, till the haemoglobin level is satisfactory. This treatment may also be given to all the patients of cancer, T. B., paralysis, arthritis and brain problem or having chronic problem and also to the children who have a deficiency of haemoglobin.

Check if the parents too have a deficiency of haemo-globin and if so ask them to take treatment.

**(26) Muscular Distrophy and similar other diseases of Brain/Neuro disorders/Mutiple Sceleriosis/Retardedness :** This disease is noticed at the end of the third year or afterwards, when there is difficulty in walking, climbing stair-cases or when the patient may start losing control of the leg muscles and may fall down frequently. Later on, it affects the shoulder muscles and once the patient is confined to wheel chair, this disease progressively paralyses the functioning of different organs of the body. Later on, the brain stops functioning and the patient dies. This disease has developed in a great proportion causing great worry. In spite of spending huge amounts every year, the disease has not been controlled so far. **However, Acupressure can play a great role in preventing and curing this disease.**

**The root causes of this disease are :**

( 1 ) Hereditary–familial.

( 2 ) Sometimes, when a woman has sex relations with more than one male, there is hormonal imbalance, which often affects her children.

( 3 ) In families having Red-Green colour blindness.

( 4 ) Disorder of the female organs. In such cases, proper care should be taken at the time of child-birth.

( 5 ) Damage to the Foetus during pregnancy, and

( 6 ) Damage to the brain of the child of less than nine months.

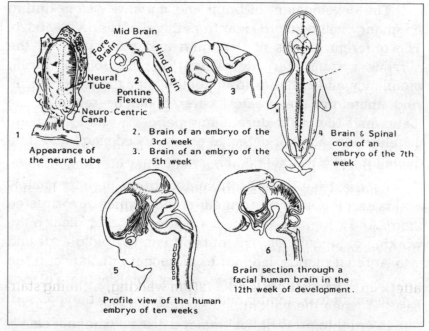

Fig. 120 : A few stages in the embroyonic development of the nervous system

In order to understand the root cause of the dreaded disease, one must know the nervous system, the telephone exchange of our body. The afferent nerves from the five senses of touch, hearing, sight, smell and taste take the messages to the brain. The computer in our brain analyses these massages and sends orders through efferent nerves to the muscles and the muscles act accordingly. Someti.. .s, we find that we receive telephone calls from outside but we cannot make a phone call to others. Sometimes, the telephone machine becomes dead even though there is no defect in it. The fault is in the telephone exchange. In the same way, the root cause of this disease is in the brain. The power of the battery becomes weak and so the electric current becomes weak and their passing is disturbed by excitatory nerves fibre due to de-polarisation of cell membrane of motor nuclei. That leads to slow and steady degeneration and there is muscular wasting in the affected muscles. *(See Chapter 2)*

The development of brain and nervous system during pregnancy will be more clear from the pictures given above. The different organs of the brain and other parts of the nervous system start developing in the foteus during pregnancy and even up to 9 months after the child's birth. And, therefore, the greatest care should be taken of the foetus and the child during this period. A slight damage develops into a major defect at an advanced stage and then damages the affected part.

As the trouble starts from the brain, it immediately affects the Pituitary and Pineal glands which are situated there. And when these glands are affected, they disturb the working of Sex glands, Thyroid and Parathyroid glands and also Adrenal glands, leading to hormonal imbalance in the body. So, at the time of this disease, the points of these glands will be found to be tender and will be paining when pressed.

In order to prevent this dreaded disease, the root cause, hereditary and damage to the brain during pregnancy should be controlled. We take great care of the earth/soil by properly ploughing, watering and cleaning it before the best quality of selected seeds are sown in it. We also take great care to see that these seeds are selected in such a way that the plant develops properly and can even resist the diseases. However, when planting a human body, no such care is taken.

Nowadays, semen is not preserved properly and allowed to be fermented till the age of 21 – 24. In the same way, most of the girls have problems of menses which clearly indicates that their ovaries are not functioning satisfactorily. Further, excess drinking of coffee, tea, liquor, smoking and even addiction to drugs have increased, thereby disturbing the metabolism of the hormones. And this imbalance of metabolism of hormones in males and females is one of the prime reasons for the improper development of the nervous system including the brain of the child to be born.

**Another reason is the improper diet, drinking, smoking and drug addiction during pregnancy.**

It is surprising that methods of preserving and cleaning the semen *(Viryashuddhi)* and the egg-ova *(Rajshuddhi)* are given in ancient Indian Health Science – *Ayurved*. The following instructions are to be carried out to arrest this disease :

( 1 ) Semen in men and Raj/Ova (रज) in women should not be disturbed/wasted through masturbation or sex play but should be allowed to ferment till the age of 21 – 24 in boys and 18 – 21 in girls.

( 2 ) Proper treatment should be taken to reduce excess heat of the body and see that menses are regular at least for 6 to 8 periods before conceiving.

( 3 ) The semen and ova (रज) can be purified and activated by drinking gold/silver/copper/iron charged water, one glass reduced from 4 glasses and also by taking Acupressure treatment every day.

( 4 ) After conceiving, the expectant mother should drink this water and take Acupressure treatment daily. This will ensure proper growth of the foetus, and its brain.

( 5 ) An expectant mother should take proper care to see that no damage is done to foetus through lack of nutritious diet, toxication by liquor, tobacco, drugs or even excess coffee and tea. And excess of all mental and physical activities should be avoided.

( 6 ) All persons suffering from venereal diseases HIV/AIDS. should be prevented from becoming parents.

( 7 ) In those families where this disease is found in the boys, their sisters have a 50/50 chance of being carriers of this disease and therefore should be put to the following tests :

(a) Serum creatine kinase estimation.

(b) quantitative electromyography,

( c ) and muscles biopsy.

And in case they are found to be carrier, they must be sterilised so that they cannot have children. They can adopt children.

**Diagnosis :**

In case the child falls down often, has a difficulty in climbing the staircase, not developing properly, has severe headache for a long time, there is no proper control in activities of organs, etc., try the following to detect this problem of Muscular Distrophy :

( 1 ) Press on patients head- three inches above both the earlobes and see if there is any hurting. See figure.

( 2 ) Press Point Nos. 1 to 5 and see if there is any hurting.

( 3 ) Press on Point No. 16 of lymph gland and find out whether there is hurting.

( 4 ) Are the calf muscles getting stiff?

In case of hurting, it could be Muscular Distrophy and/or Brains

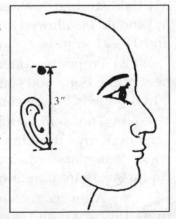

Fig. 121

problem. In case the hurting is observed on Point No. 16 and 1 to 5 it could be a tumour in the brain. DO NOT PANIC.

**Treatment :** For those patients who are already affected by this disease, the following treatment will greatly assist them to control these and similar other diseases of the brain and the nervous system : i. e. retardedness/multiple sceleriosis, etc.

( 1 ) High powered–concentrated gold/silver/copper/ iron charged water to be given as under :

$\frac{1}{2}$ glass reduced from 8 glasses for 8 days.

1 glass reduced from 8 glasses for 8 days.

2 glasses reduced from 8 glasses to be given till recovery and 3 months afterwards.

1 glass reduced from 2 glasses for a long time afterwards. This treatment will give a push to the brain and motor nuclei and start their functions.

( 2 ) Acupressure treatment of 2 minutes 3 times a day to be given to Point Nos. 1 to 6, 11 to 15, 25, 28 and 38.

( 3 ) Treatment on webs and back of palms twice a day will be useful to relieve any nervous tension and correct any impairment to them. Also it will tone them up.

( 4 ) Health drink/powder to be given twice a day. One teaspoon Health powder can be added to 1 cup of green juice.

( 5 ) Green juices of leafy vegetables and honey is to be freely given 2 to 4 cups a day.

( 6 ) Fresh fruit juices–2 to 3 glasses to be given daily.

( 7 ) Blue light to be given for 15 minutes each on the head and on the spinal cord and affected parts twice a day. (Refer page 134 and 202)

( 8 ) Kapalbhati and Bhastrika–see page 117.

( 9 ) Pranayam–see page 111/112.

(10) Rub the soles of the patient for 5 + 5 minutes in the morning and evening till the soles are warmer than the head.

**Case Study :** *A lady brought her eight year handsome son, who was developing well since birth. But after his seventh birthday, he started finding it difficult in climbing steps of a staircase and within next six months it developed to such an extent that he was unable to climb the staircase. On examination, it was found to be an obvious case of Muscular Distrophy. Mother was asked to give treatment. After four months, she came with a complaint that her son was allright but had become naughty and would go down in the lift and come running on the staircase all the way upto sixth floor, where they were residing. What a good news it was!*

**(27) Polio :** This is due to virus infection in the motor nuclei of brain stem and in the gray matter of the spinal cord and paralysis of the connected muscles.

( 1 ) Give treatment as mentioned under 26 mentioned above.

( 2 ) Give vapour treatment or hot pack treatment on the affected part for one month.

( 3 ) Afterwards, give hot and cold packs alternately for 10 minutes twice a day.

( 4 ) After this, dry up the affected parts and rub oil on them as mentioned on page 201.

( 5 ) First give red light for 4 to 5 minutes on the affected parts (not on head) and then blue light for 8 to 10 minutes on the affected parts + on head – twice a day.

( 6 ) Practise sun Pranayam, Kapal Bhati and Bhastrika as much as possible.

If the treatment is given within 3 months, it is totally cured. Even if the treatment is tried later, it gives good result and reduces the defect.

**(28) Meningitis :** This is due to congestion of water in the brain.

( 1 ) Please give the patient full bed rest.

( 2 ) All treatments as mentioned under 26 to be given.

(3) Give brain wash as mentioned on page 264 on 1st, 5th & 10th day only. That will give 20 to 30 sneezings.

(4) Do not worry about fever. Only keep it under control with cold packs.

**Caution :** In hospitals fluid is extracted from the top of head. Many times, this disturbs the Pineal gland and thereby pituitary and other glands, which leads to malfunctioning of some organs and leads to early awakening of sex desire, leading to juvenile delinquency.

**(29) Parkinson's Disease :** Shivering of any part of the body – (mostly hands) : This is due to hypertension. Sometimes the nerve endings in the brain break down. And control over hands, and later on, over other parts of the body becomes weak and so hands start shivering. This is called Parkinson's disease. As the damage is in the brain, all the treatmen˙ mentioned above for brain under (26) is necessary. Moreover, give the treatment for nervous tension as mentioned on pages 221 – 222 plus treatment as per fig. 115 is also necessary. Just within 2/3 months, you will get amazing results.

**Case Study :** *One surgeon, M. S. Doctor of Mumbai was specialising in operations of the children. He suffered from this problem and so had to stop doing operations. He started this treatment. Within four months, he started doing operations again.*

**(30) Mental Breakdown/Depression and Madness :** All treatments as mentioned in 26 plus as mentioned under 13.

**(31) Coma :** When the motor neuron in the brain is damaged, one goes into coma and remains unconscious sometimes even for six months before death. In order to start the stopped engine of a car, sometimes it is necessary to give it a push. The same way if such a push is given to brain-motor neuron, it starts functioning and the patient becomes conscious.

To do so do the following :

( 1 ) Give the patient every day 1 oz (30 ml) of concentrated gold/silver/pure diamonds (1 to 2 carat) charged water reduced from 32 oz (2 litre) till the patient becomes conscious.

( 2 ) Give the treatment on Point No. 1 to 5 and 36 for 2 minutes each in the morning and evening.

( 3 ) Give the treatment on both the points above the earlobes as per fig. 115 – for 2 minutes on each point – in the morning and in the evening.

( 4 ) Rub nylon brush or ghee in the soles of the legs for 5 minutes on each sole, twice a day.

( 5 ) Give blue light on the head for 5 to 6 minutes twice daily.

Continue all these treatments till the patient becomes conscious, Then, follow the treatment as given under (26) page 249. Also find out the root cause and give treatment accordingly.

The above treatment has been tried on several patients – even when they were in coma for more than six months. In all such cases, the patient has not only regained consciousness but become normal.

In all cases of serious and chronic diseases also combine the treatment shown in chapters 6, 7, 8 and 9 for faster recovery.

The cure achieved as a result of this treatment is not temporary but of lasting nature. The organ starts functioning normally and will continue as long as the laws of Nature are observed. You will also note that Nature helps us to cure the diseases if we give it time to cure us. And Acupressure treatment helps Nature – (our body) – to get rid of the disease faster. And thereafter, with regular treatment, health could be maintained.

In case of contagious diseases, it is advisable to keep the patient isolated. At least, keep the children away from such a patient. Wash his clothes and utensils separately and maintain cleanliness.

Please note that all the diseases, whatever may be their names, are related to the functioning organs of the body. Therefore, for treating any disease, not named here, the root cause and the organ affected must be found out and treatment should be given on the point corresponding to that particular organ. For cure of all dreaded diseases like common cold Asthma, Cataract, Thalesemmia and HIV/AIDS, read author's Book "Health in Your Hands : Volume 2."

Please note that any disease except Death is curable. And Death is a MUST for every living being. Do not be afraid of Death. It is the door through which everybody has to pass to enter a new world. Death is like a kind mother who takes away this old body, old clothes and gives us new clothes i. e. new body – a new life.

———

# CHAPTER 16

# INSTRUCTIONS TO
# THE PRACTITIONERS

( 1 ) The practitioners of the Acupressure Therapy must study Physiology thoroughly so that he/she becomes well conversant with the functioning of the body. This will help them to diagnose the root cause of a disease properly.

( 2 ) In case of any problem, just check up the Solar Plexus, and set it right if it is not in order (see page 65). Secondly, see that the network of nerves passing through the spinal cord is in order. Otherwise, correct it as shown in fig. 83.

( 3 ) He/she should confine the total treatment to not more than five minutes on the first three days.

( 4 ) Subsequently, longer treatment (2 to 3 minutes) on each point is possible on the soles but do not give more than 2 minutes treatment on any one point of the palms.

( 5 ) After other points are treated, treatment must be given on Point No. 26 of the kidney on both the palms or soles because the toxins thrown out by the other organs of the body will come to the kidneys. So, the kidneys must be activated to throw out these poisons/toxins from the body.

( 6 ) In case there is pain on more than 3 points on the palm or sole, it is a clear sign that the life battery has become weak. So, in such cases and in cases of chronic diseases, the patient must be advised to drink lukewarm copper/silver/ gold charged water and health drink at least 2 to 3 times during the day. Moreover, light food and longer hours of sleep are a must. This will help the patient to recharge and empower his life battery and he will get cured fast.

( 7 ) For the patients suffering from chronic diseases or confined to bed, feel their endocrine glands (Pituitary, Pineal,

Thyroid, Adrenal, Pancreas, Sex glands). If you observe that there is pain in at least 2 of these glands, it means that these glands are also to be treated first. But be careful not to treat any of these glands for more than one minute on the first day. Only after the 3rd treatment if the pain continues, about 2 minutes treatment can be given for these glands, 3 times a day on the palms or 4 to 6 minutes on the soles.

(8) The practitioners must never jump upon any Diagnosis. Please study all angles, symptoms, etc. and postpone Diagnosis for next sitting. But start general treatment and charged water 2 glasses reduced from four glasses.

The practitioners must also study other therapies like Chromotherapy, Naturopathy and Biochemic medicines, etc. as mentioned in this book and also use these therapies wherever necessary to give faster relief to the patients.

**Magnet and Acupressure :** When Acupressure treatment is given, because of flow of Bio-electricity, magnetic field in the body becomes normal. Therefore, it is not advised to combine magnetic treatment. At least the use of high power or electric magnets should be avoided, when Acupressure treatment is given.

**Last but not the least, confidence must be created in the patient that Nature is very kind and the body is capable of curing all diseases and that Acupressure therapy hastens the process of healing.** Thereafter, the treatment given on all the points will hasten the process of healing.

The practitioner should teach this therapy to the patient, so that the patient can treat himself without the help of others.

The practitioner must bear in mind that this is a God-given therapy, installed in our body and therefore he can definitely cure the patients by pressing on the tender spots either in palms or soles. A blind or even an invalid person can easily master this art of healing and can earn his bread with dignity.

# CHAPTER 17

# TEN MINUTES A DAY TO KEEP
# THE DISEASE AWAY

Daily treatment of Acupressure is to be taken on the two palms and/or the two soles :

You must have observed that all the points on two palms are up to 1 inch below the wrists and upto one inch around the ankles. So, without worrying about where the different points are located, just go on pressing both the palms **OR** soles/(front and back) for 5 minutes each.

For those above 40, two minutes pressure on one inch circle between the wrist and the elbow of the right hand is to be taken as shown in fig. 81. This treatment can be taken at any time in any position and should be made a part of one's daily routine. Before taking this treatment, check the Solar Plexus and correct it, if necessary.

Over and above this treatment, the following exercises may be done for maintaining good health, strengthening the endocrine glands and keeping the body fit and supple.

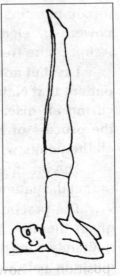

**( 1 ) Spot jogging :** Running at one spot. Start with 1 minute daily and reach 2 to 3 minutes.

**( 2 ) Sarvangasan :** Lie down on the back, lift the legs straight up and then support the body with your hands till you come to the position as shown in the figure. It is useful to throat, head and the full body through proper blood circulation.

Fig. 122

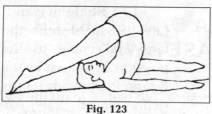

Fig. 123

**(3) Halasan :** Lie down on the back, take the stretched legs behind to touch the ground as shown in the figure. Useful to spine and digestive organs and abdomen.

**(4) Padpaschimottanasan :** Sit with stretched legs, bend forward, touch the toes with the finger-tips, bend still further till you reach the positions as shown in the figure. Later on, try to touch the knees, with the forehead. Useful to digestive organs and the spine.

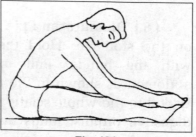

Fig. 124

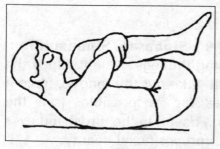

Fig. 125

**(5) Pavanmuktasan :** Lie down, on your back. Bend the legs and bring them inside, clasp them with the hands. Bring the head up to touch the knees as shown in the figure. Cures gas trouble.

**(6) Bhujangasan :** Lie on the stomach, pull the hands below the shoulders. Raise your head and the trunk from the front till you come to the position as shown in the figure. Useful to digestive organs and the spine.

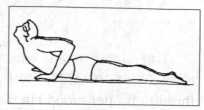

Fig. 126

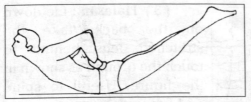

Fig. 127

**( 7 ) Shalabhasan :** Lift the head and the legs and come to the position as shown in the figure. Place your hands (with closed fists) on your hips. Useful to digestive organs, the spine and the abdomen.

**( 8 ) Dhanurasan :** Lie down on the stomach. Hold the legs with the hands. Pull up the abdomen as shown in the figure. Useful to the whole sciatic nerve, digestive organs, lungs and the abdomen.

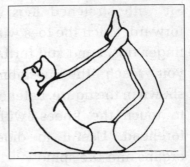

Fig. 128

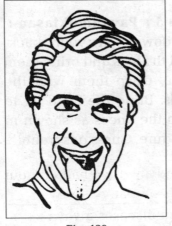

Fig. 129

**( 9 ) Sinhasan/Sinhamudra :** Bending the legs sit tight. Open the mouth, take out the tongue, force it out as far as possible. (see the figure.) Useful to the throat and eyes and improves facial beauty.

**(10)** Stand erect keeping a distance of 12 inches between the two legs. Raise the hands as per fig. 130. Then twist to the left as fast as possible, giving a jerk. Come to the above position. Twist to the right as fast as possible. Come back. Repeat 10 times. This exercise is very helpful for activating the spleen and the liver.

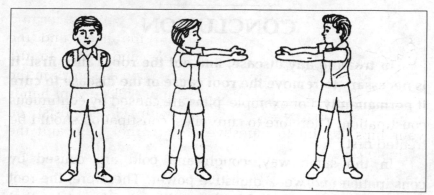

**Fig. 130**

In the beginning, all the positions shown may not be mastered. But with practice, one will be able to master each position.

**Duration of all these asans :** Starting with 10 seconds reach upto 1 minute for each asan/position.

**Breathing :** Normal.

**Dress :** As light and loose as possible. Cotton dress is preferable.

**Effect :** All these exercises help proper digestion, blood circulation, proper oxygenation, proper functioning of the endocrine glands, and add to the suppleness of the body.

**Net result :** Regular exercises would keep the body healthy and fit. Sinhasan is very good for throat and facial beauty. People of any age can do these 'asans'.

**Pranayam :** This can be practised any time half an hour before meals and 3 hours after meals and anywhere.

**Ten minutes a day and keep the diseases away :**

Acupressure can be practised at any time during the day-while lying down, sitting and standing while travelling or in office and so special time is required.

And only for doing all those 'asans' you require only ten minutes. Thus, only ten minutes a day are enough to keep the diseases away.

# CHAPTER 18

# CONCLUSION

**In treating any disease, find out the root cause first. It is necessary to remove the root cause of the disease to cure it permanently.** For example, piles are caused by continuous constipation. Therefore to cure piles, constipation should be treated first.

In the same way, cough and cold are caused by constipation and weak digestive power. Therefore, the root causes should be removed when taking treatment for that particular disease.

**Mind :** Mind has a great control over our body. A happy (healthy) mind in a healthy body is the goal to be attained.

Happiness of mind can be achieved by stopping all unnecessary worries. It will be observed that in Nature, nobody worries for future. If a list is made of all the worries, it will be found that most of them are unnecessary and could be easily avoided.

It has been observed that in most of the psychological problems, the endocrine glands are disturbed and not corrected afterwards. In such cases, treatment on all the endocrine glands would prove highly beneficial.

Secondly, everybody should take interest in others and in literature, music, art, sports, etc. (fine arts)

The third and the most important point is :

To love all beings and be friendly with them :

To forgive them all and ask them to forgive you.

**Please note that :**

To give is Divine.

To earn a living honestly is Human.

To snatch others' property and cause pain to others in body, by words or even mentally is a sin.

We all are born as Humans. Let's try to be Humane and Divine.

When Mother Nature has provided us with such a simple and easy treatment to cure diseases and even to avoid them, we all must follow the instructions given by her. These Therapies only help Nature to cure us. Let us not ignore Nature in our mad pursuit of science.

**This Nature's 'DO IT YOURSELF' ACUPRESSURE Therapy itself is a science and not a matter of belief.**

Dear reader, you know that this treatment does not cost you any money. Moreover, it is harmless as it has no side effects. Therefore, as a sensible person craving for good health, which is our **birthright,** try this therapy sincerely and regularly for at least 15 days and observe its wonderful and amazing results. Thus, you will become your own Doctor and a firm believer in "YOUR HEALTH IS IN YOUR HANDS." At the time of pressing your palms or soles, please thank the Great Power which has installed this wonderful system of self-cure in our body.

---

## DO THIS DAILY

1. Press your two palms each for 5 minutes – on front and back.

2. If over 40 years, press for 2 minutes the middle of right arm (see fig. 81 on page 162).

3. Then on all points where it pains, give treatment 3 times a day for 2/2 minutes on each point like pumping.

4. In the evening, while sitting in a chair, roll your soles of the legs on a roller. see fig. 69 on page 125.

5. Make a habit of drinking :
   ( 1 ) One glass of hot water, preferably charged water as the first thing in the morning.
   ( 2 ) Drink one cup of green juice adding 1 teaspoon of health powder and 1 tablespoon of honey to it.
   ( 3 ) Drink one glass of fresh fruit juice.

6. Correct the Solar Plexus and avoid constipation.

---

## USEFUL HINTS

### ( 1 ) For increasing heat in the body :

( a ) Drink $\frac{1}{2}$ glass of hot water every 30 minutes till you feel fresh.

( b ) **Take the following with hot water :** $\frac{1}{2}$ teaspoon of Turmeric powder+$\frac{1}{2}$ teaspoon of ground Bishop's seeds (अजवाईन) & OR $\frac{1}{2}$ teaspoon of Mahasudarshan powder.

( c ) Rub the soles with soft nylon brush (used for washing clothes) 5 to 10 minutes – three times a day, till the soles are warmer than the head.

### ( 2 ) For removing excess heat from the body :

( a ) Take as first thing in the morning 1 teaspoonful of haritki churna (harde powder – powder of terminalia chebula retz)+$\frac{1}{2}$ teaspoon of sugar for 8 to 10 days continuously, then twice a week. This will also keep the bowels clean.

( b ) Soak powder of 15 black pepper (काली मरी)+2 tea-spoonful of (preferably crystal) sugar in $1\frac{1}{2}$ glass of water. Blend them and sip all as first thing in morning for 10 days. After 10 days, add 5 almonds to the blending and drink it for further 10 days. This is very useful even in jaundice, psirosis, sunstroke, etc.

( c ) Take 5 black pepper (काली मिर्च)+10/12 black raisins (काली द्राक्ष) +1 teaspoon of saunf (सौंप). Soak them in a glass of water in the evening. Next day, blend them and drink it in the afternoon. A useful drink in summer.

( d ) Take an equal quantity of cumin seed powder (जीरा), black pepper (काली मिर्च), saunf (सौंप), amla powder (आमला), crystal sugar (मीसरी), and ginger powder (सुंठ). Grind them into powder and keep it in a bottle. Take 1 teaspoonful of this powder with water in the morning and evening.

**( 3 ) For Tonsils :** Mix 2 drops of glycerine tanic acid with $\frac{1}{2}$ teaspoonful of turmeric powder (हलदी). Apply it on both the tonsils inside the throat and then gargle with lukewarm salted water. Do this two to three times a day.

**( 4 ) Bleeding or pain in gums :** Massage the above mentioned mixture of glycerine tanic acid and turmeric powder on the gums and then gargle with lukewarm salted water. Then massage edible oil preferably castor oil on gums.

**( 5 ) Earache and pus :** Put 2 drops of Hydrogen Peroxide in the ears. Clean the foams and then put ear drops.

**( 6 ) To activate kidney :** Over and above giving Acupressure treatment for 2 minutes three times a day on Point No. 26 of the kidney, drink 1 cup of black tea. (Put 1 cup of water to boil; put in it 1 teaspoonful of any leaf tea). Boil till the water is reduced to $\frac{1}{2}$ a cup. Filter it and add $\frac{1}{2}$ a cup of water; drink as first thing in the morning for 12 to 15 days till the first urine of morning becomes clear and odourless.

If possible, drink daily silver charged water 2 glasses reduced from 8 glasses. For prevention of any kidney problem, this treatment may be tried once a year. With this treatment, dialysis and even operations for kidney transplantations are prevented.

**( 7 ) To cure Rashes :** Add 2 teaspoonful of turmeric powder (हलदी) + 2 teaspoonful of grounded bishop's seeds (अजवाईन) + 2 teaspoonfuls of sugar in 4 glasses of water. Boil it and reduce it to two glasses. Drink one glass of such water the first thing in the morning and the other glass in the evening before sunset. Within 2 to 3 days, rashes will be cured.

**( 8 ) For Diabetes :** Over and above taking treatment on all endocrine glands for 2/2 minutes 3 times a day;

(i) Drink 2 glasses of gold/silver/copper/iron charged water–reduced from 4 glasses of water.

(ii) Drink $\frac{1}{2}$ a cup of juice of corriander leaves (कोथमीर – हरा धनीया) as first thing in the morning for 30/40 days till sugar level has come to normal.

**( 9 ) Pain reliever :** For all types of pain, the following treatment gives instant but **temporary** relief. Take 1 tea-spoonful of ordinary salt. Heat it in a pan till it becomes brown/gray. Put 1 to 2 grains (a little) of it on tongue/every fifteen minutes till the pain subsides but limit it to 3 to 4 times only.

If this salt is taken at night, it causes sleep. (for Insomnia)

**Be careful not to take this salt in excess or form the habit of taking it.**

**(10) To purify blood :** For 30 days, drink the juice of the following as first thing in the morning :

21 leaves with the stalk of bitter neem. (Azadi racta Indica)

21 leaves with the stalk of tulsi. (Holi Basil)

21 (7 × 3) leaves with the stalk of bilipatra (Aegle Mar)

Honey can be added to the juice.

(Only if such leaves are not available, powder of same can be used OR tinctures of the same duly mixed will be available at Homeopathic/ Pharmacy shops. Take 5 drops of this mixed tincture in half a cup of lukewarm water in the morning and evening.)

**(11) Head–Brain Wash :** In case of severe headache, congestion of sinus or brain problem, the following powder is very useful for **instant** but **short term** relief.

**How to prepare :** Take kayfal 70 % (कायफल). (If not available – take black pepper), cardamom 20 % (एलायची), and saffron 10 % (केशर). Grind them into very fine powder and keep it in a bottle. Do not worry if saffron is not added. In that case 80 % of kayfal powder + 20 % of cardamom powder will give good result.

**How to use :** Take a little of this powder and inhale it like snuff deeply into one nostril – while closing the other one and then into another nostril, keeping the first one closed. There will be watering from the nose and the eyes and heavy sneezing for about 10 to 30 times. Do not worry if the mucus coming out is reddish. Repeat, if necessary. But only TWICE a week, but not for more than 2 weeks.

**(12) How to create cooling effect in the body :** Open the mouth, put out the tongue and draw in (inhale) air through the mouth. Close the mouth. And exhale through nose after retaining the inhaled air as long as possible. Repeat 15/25 times. You will immediately feel cool. This method is called 'SHITALI' (शितलि) in Yoga and found to be very useful in summer, sunstroke, fever or whenever cooling effect is necessary.

# OTHER USEFUL REFERENCES

## Clarification of words/terms for all Foreigners/Non Indians

| | |
|---|---|
| Rishis | = Ancient Yogis-saints |
| Injection | = shot |
| Peg | = short |
| Gram flour | = flour of a pulse called gram / basin |
| Sudarshan Powder (सुदर्शन चुर्ण) | = A bitter Ayurvedic Powder |
| Harde/Haritki (हरडे / हरितकी चुर्ण) | = Powder of Terminalia Chebula Retz-an Ayurvedic medicine |
| Kayfal (कायफल) | = N. O. Myricacae |
| Bilipatra (बिलीपत्र) | = Aegle Mar |
| Neem (नीम) | = Azadiracta Indica |
| Tulsi (श्यामतूलसी) | = Ocimum centum – Holy Basil |
| Amla (आमला) | = Embalica – an India fruit (containing concentrated vitamin C) |
| Nux Vomica \| Thuja | = Homeopathic medicines |
| Cal. Phos + Cal. Fl. + Kali Phos + Nat. Mur + Kali Iodide | = Biochemic medicines |

(All Homeopathic & Biochemic medicines are available in any Homeopathic Drug Store/Pharmacy).

# READY RECKONER – INDEX

| Diseases/Troubles | Points | Page |
|---|---|---|
| 6. Polio | (All points twice daily + copper/silver/ gold charged water) | ... 250 |
| 7. Smallpox/Chickenpox | (22, 23, 28 & 38) | ... 209 |
| 8. Teething troubles | (All points + Calcium) | ... 184 |
| 9. Thalesemmia | — | ... 243 |
| 10. Wetting the bed | — | ... 186 |
| 11. Whooping Cough | (1 to 7, 30, 34 & 38 + treatment on Page 79) | ... 179 |
| Cancer | — | ... 232 |
| Cholesterol | — | ... 212 |
| Coma | — | ... 251 |
| Constipation | — | ... 222 |
| Cough & Cold | (1 to 7, 30 & 34) | ... 176 |
| Cold due to heat | — | ... 174 |
| Corn | — | ... 195 |
| Deafness/dumbness | (31) | ... 192 |
| Diabetes | (25 & 26) | ... 213 |
| Dizziness & severe pain in Sinus | — | ... 194 |
| Dumbness | (31) | ... 193 |
| Dysentery/Vomitting | (19, 20, 23, 25, 27 & 38) | ... 180 |
| Ear Pain & Puss | (31 & 16) | ... 192 |
| Emergency Elephantiasis/Filariasis | — | ... 229 |
| Epilepsy – Fits | (All points + Press earlobes) | ... 184 |
| Eosinophilia | — | ... 219 |
| Excess of Biles (Pitt) | — | ... 183 |
| Eyes – Cataract/Tracoma | (35) | ... 190 |
| Optic nerve | back of palms | ... 190 |
| Fever due to cold (Flu) or Bronchitis | (1 to 7, 30 & 34) | ... 178 |
| Fever due to Malaria | (1 to 7, 30, 34 & 37) | ... 178 |

# NEW CONCEPT ABOUT ENERGY

The therapies of Acupressure, Acupuncture, Shiatsu, etc. are based on the principle of bio-electricity. Moreover, E.E.G. and E.C.G. also prove the existence of electricity flowing in the body, So, to function properly, the human body requires electricity with equal positive and negative charge. It has been proved that excess of positive electricity creates excess of heat in the body – leading to many problems of hyperacidity – sluggish liver, damage to the brain. etc. and other diseases. Excess of negative electricity leads to excess of water content in the body, reducing the digestion power in the body. That is why the food we take should be as far as possible balanced in positive and negative electric charges.

It is a well-known fact of science that energy cannot be created, it can only be transformed. Now due to combustion of hydrogen gas, the sun has become a tremendous powerhouse of energy. This is received on the earth in the form of sunlight which not only gives us light and heat but also electric energy. All the vegetation, fruits, crops, etc. is there only because of the sun. The cereals, pulses go on collecting this solar energy for 30 to 45 days after the bush has developed. And when this staple food is consumed, it is converted into energy in our body. In the same way, the fruits gather this solar energy and grow bigger and ripen and when eaten they give good amount of nutrition, Likewise, this solar energy is collected by the grass and leaves. The thicker the leaves, the more is solar energy and medicinal value they have. Moreover, green grass and leaves are easily digestible and contain in them equal quantity of positive and negative electricity. The mammals like goat, cow, buffalo and camel consume green grass and leaves and convert the hidden energy into nutritious milk. Animals like the horse, the rhinoceros and the elephant live only on this vegetation and are considered to be the strongest. Now, we can tap this abundant and free energy for our body. It is true that we cannot eat large quantities of grass and vegetation; but the extract of leaves, grass and of all non-poisonous vegetation can be consumed easily. It is digestible and it gives the human body all types of salts, minerals, vitamin C and a good amount of energy.

In case of a dreaded disease like cancer, the main problem often is loss of weight and stamina because more cells die every day than are created new in the body. In all types of cancer, the patients are kept on a special diet of :

( 1 ) 4 to 5 cups of green juice extracted out of all types of leafy vegetables, cabbage, carrots, etc. adding thereto honey.

( 2 ) 2 glasses of fruit juice.

( 3 ) Plenty of green salads + sprouted pulses and after 15 days, 8 to 10 oz of curds.

And surprisingly, these patients gain weight of about 3 to 5 lbs per month, get more stamina and also their disease is cured.

Similarly, in all chronic cases and brain problems, the patients are kept on the above diet and the results are astounding. This only proves the great amount of energy and medicinal value this green juice has.

Every year, lots of these leaves ripen and fall down and are wasted. These leaves can be used to get their extract. Even the dried leaves can be soaked in water for two hours and their extract can be taken. Moreover, it is possible to grow 20 to 24 crops of such vegetation in a year. The waste of these green leaves can be used as fodder for the animals and can be used as a wet pack for skin problems. Thus, there will be full utilisation of the leaves.

Honey is a great source of solar energy and has great medicinal value, when it is added to the green juice in the proportion of 1 tablespoon to one cup of green juice, it becomes a perfect food, is easily digestible and is very quickly transformed into blood.

Secondly, after the body is fully developed by the age of 18-21, what the human body requires is enough electric energy to maintain it in such a condition that the body remains energetic and is capable of doing all the required work and of enjoying life fully. Therefore, from the age of 20 onwards, food intake should be reduced gradually and after the age of 60, the intake of food should be brought down to the minimum. Our diet should be supplemented more and more with green juice, honey and fruits. Moreover, if everybody carries out the experiment shown in this book to find out which eatables/drinks are suitable to his body and eats accordingly, the total requirement of food will be minimised to a great extent.

It may be noted that through the experiments carried out in China and Japan it has been found out that if one develops a practice of eating preparations of only one cereal like rice or wheat or pulses without any salt or spices and milk, vegetables or fruits, etc. and stays on such diet for 12 days twice a year, his body acquires the proper balance of positive and negative electricity and becomes so immune as to resist even the nuclear radiation. Afterwards, if a balanced diet consisting of 65 % of staple food + 35 % of milk and its products; oils, fruits, vegetables, etc. are taken with minimum of spices; the body remains healthy and energetic throughout life. This is also amply proved by Jains in India. They do a penance of 9 days twice a year. They take preparations of rice on the first day, wheat on the second day, gram on the third day, Chinese peas i. e. Mung, on the fourth day; black Udada on the fifth day and only rice on the remaining four days. They have been doing this for thousands of years. Sometimes, some one performs such penance (called आयंबिल) for 500 days. It has been observed that such a person does not suffer from any disease for want of nutrition or vitamins. This is only because he consumes food which has equal quantum of positive and negative electricity in it. Moreover, he takes such food only once a day and boiled water during the day. This clearly proves that the human body can stay healthy and capable of doing the daily chores with the minimum of food. This fact is also proved by Mahatma Gandhiji, Shri Vinoba Bhave, Morarji Desai and many others. Moreover, it also proves that there is no necessity of eating meat, fish, eggs, etc. to get more energy.

If all the people gradually follow this principle of reducing the food intake and supplementing it with green juice, fruits, etc., there will be enough food available on the earth and there will not be any more famine. Moreover, the body will remain healthy and most of the problems of indigestion, overweight, etc. will be controlled automatically. It may be noted that just by consuming more juice of GREEN, people will become EVERGREEN.

# WHAT THE PEOPLE SAY ABOUT THIS BOOK

*"Health in Your Hands"* is found to be very useful. The language is simple and all the suggestions are practical and so one can become the practitioner of Acupressure only by just reading it thoroughly. It is a boon to the mankind."

Thousands of readers not only in India but all over the World say thus.

**What the Medical Practitioners say about this book :**

"Your book enabled me to cure my twenty year old constipation within just 2 days."

*– Dr Sat Paul Singh, Professor of Punjab University, Patiala.*

"Tata Memorial Hospital, Mumbai discharged my brother as they found his Cancer of throat to be incurable. I consulted Sri Devendra Vora and followed the instructions given in the book. My brother resumed duty within 45 days."

*– Dr R. K. Mehta, a Homeopath, Mumbai.*

"My wife was losing weight and stamina and the disease was not diagnosed. Sri Vora made a correct Diagnosis and she started treatment as per the book. She gained weight and stamina and within 60 days she fully recovered."

*– Dr Suresh Gandhi, M. D., Porbundar.*

"I have found your book most interesting and valuable. We would like you to conduct a course of Acupressure in our institute."

*– Dr (Mrs) Radha, Rest-New Era Development Institute, Panchgani.*

"I have just read your book "Health in Your Hands." This is one of the finest books, I have read on Reflexology. I am a Doctor in South Africa, practising Acupressure."

*– Dr S. Isseri (MB chb.) D. Sc., F.R.C.S.*

"On the basis of your book, I had spread health to the people of Mauritius and now I am spreading health to the people of Fiji. My blessings and congratulations for writing this book for the benefit of the mankind."

*– Swami Sanjivani Anand, Suva-Fiji.*

*"The useful book is now revised to make it more useful."*

*"Readers are requested to express their views to the press-so many patients like them can benefit from this therapy."*

# ACKNOWLEDGEMENT WITH RESPECTS TO

| | |
|---|---|
| Kind Mother Nature | Who has installed this wonderful system in our body. |
| Ancient unknown sages Known and Unknown | Who found this Therapy |
| Ayurved Experts | Who developed this Therapy |
| Unknown Red Indians and all those unknown races | Who preserved this Therapy |
| Dr William Fritzerald, U. S. A. | Who made research in the 20th century and put this Therapy before the world. |
| Mrs Mildred Carter, U. S. A. | "Reflexology-Foot and Hand" |
| All other Naturopaths | Who made research and developed this Therapy |
| Dr Rohit Oza, India | "Children's Diseases" |
| Mr Augustus Muller | "Bio-chemic Medicines" |
| Mr Sadashiv P. Nimbalkar | "Arogya Sathi Yoga" |
| Mr Pedro Chan | "Finger Acupressure" |
| Dr Harshad Pandya | For constant inspiration, guidance and for suggesting appropriate name for this book |
| Dr Dipak Kamdar, Ph. D. | For useful hints and cover photograph |
| All people, friends and relatives | For accepting this Therapy and giving inspiration |
| World Health Organisation, Geneva | For giving kind attention to this Therapy |
| Dr Roger Dalet | "Relief from Pain with Finger Massage" |
| Dr V. G. Rele | "Human Mind Power" |
| Dr Lord Brain & Dr John Walton | "Diseases of Nervous System" |
| Dr Richard Snail | "Clinical Neuro-Anatomy" |
| Dr J. Robert McClintic | "Physiology of the Human Body" |
| Swedish Doctors | "A Child is Born" |
| Swami Shivananda Saraswati | "Yogic Therapy" |
| Swami Yogeswaranand Saraswati | Science of Soul" |

| | |
|---|---|
| Sri B. P. Chainani, Mumbai | For treatment of Sciatic Nerve, Pyeletis and many useful hints. |
| Sri Sumanlal Shah, Kolkata | Chennai |
| Dr Chandra Sekhar Thakur, Ayurvedacharya, Mumbai | Polarisation of electricity and elements of tastes. |
| Sri G. S. Sharma Yogacharya, Mumbai | Sadhana of Ohm and useful hints |
| Dr G. K. Thakkar, Mumbai | Urine Therapy |
| Prof Ramesh Amin, Ahmedabad | Useful hints about first two chapters and translating the first two chapters in Gujarati |
| M/s Gala Publishers Mumbai | For publishing this book in India in English – Hindi – Marathi & Gujarati & Bengali languages at concessional rates. |
| Sri Deepak Idnani, Mumbai | My 25 years old student who has found out points of optic nerve. |
| Prof Dr Sir Anton Jayasuria of Open International University for Alternate Medicines, Colombo-Sri Lanka | For awarding honorary degree of M. D. to me for this book & Merit Medal for Research in Cancer and appointing me as a visiting Professor for M.D's Course. |

And I am grateful to many friends and all the patients who have tried this therapy and encouraged me with the results.

And also to Rigved, Ramayana, Mahabharata, Bhagwat, Books on Jainism, Bible, Koran and other religious scriptures for inspiration and new light on our body.

---

**Published by**   Navneet Publications (India) Ltd., Dantali, Gujarat.
**Printed by**     Navneet Publications (India) Ltd., Dantali, Gujarat.

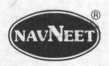

# HEALTH IN YOUR HANDS

## Volume 1

( Based on Acupressure and other Natural Therapies )

Simple Practical Way to Perfect Health

**(This book is also available in Hindi, Marathi, Bengali & Gujarati)**

by

**DEVENDRA VORA,** M.D. (Honorary)

Thirty Edition

**NAVNEET PUBLICATIONS (INDIA) LIMITED**

| **Navneet House** | **Navneet Bhavan** |
|---|---|
| Gurukul Road, Memnagar, | Bhavani Shankar Road, |
| Ahmadabad–380 052. | Dadar, Mumbai–400 028. |
| Phone : 5530 5000 | Phone : 5662 6565 |

**DHANLAL BROTHERS DISTRIBUTORS**

70, Princess Street, Mumbai–400 002.

Phone : 2201 7027

Visit us at : www.navneet.com

G 4500

e-mail : npil@navneet.com

**Price : Rs. 70.00**

(Concessional rate for India only)

Write to: **Dr. Devendra VORA**

**(Only in Hindi or English or Gujarati)**

C/7, Vasant Kunj, North Avenue,

Santacruz (W), Mumbai – 400 054.

Phone: 2649 1564

Only between 8.00 to 10.00 A.M.

& 5.00 to 8.00 P.M.

E-mail: doctordevendra@vsnl.net

For Personal Guidance Contact Dr. Devendra Vora at

## ACUPRESSURE CENTRES

**1) SANTACRUZ (West):**
SMT B C J HOSPITAL ACUP. CENTRE
(Asha Parekh S & M Ward), S. V. Rd.,
Santacruz (W), Mumbai – 400 054.

**Days/Timings:**
Wednesdays  9.00 a.m. to 10.30 a.m.
Saturdays     4.30 p.m. to  6.00 p.m.

**2) KHAR (West):**
THE KHAR RESIDENTS' ASSOCN. (Regd.)
Kamalabai Nimbkar Library,
Nr. Madhu Park, Khar (West),
Mumbai – 400 052.

**Days/Timings:**
Sundays      9.00 a.m. to. 11.00 a.m.
Thursdays    4.00 p.m. to  6.00 p.m.

**3) GHATKOPAR (West):**
SARVODAYA HOSP. ACUP. CENTRE
LBS Marg, Ghatkopar (W),
Mumbai – 400 086

**Days/Timings:**
Saturdays 9.00 a.m. to 10.30 a.m.
Tuesdays  9.00 a.m. to 10.30 a.m.

**4) CHEMBUR:**
MEDICAL RELIEF CENTRE
Shree Chembur Jain Sangh,
Opp. Jain Mandir, Chembur,
Mumbai – 400 071.

**Days/Timings:**
Mondays 4.00 p.m. to 6.00 p.m.
Fridays  4.00 p.m. to 6.00 p.m.

Dr. Devendra Vora conducts Training Course of
"BE A DOCTOR IN 12 HOURS" Based on his Bestseller
books "HEALTH IN YOUR HANDS – VOLUME I & II".
Any Organization/University who desire to arrange such
Training Seminar may contact at the above address.